The Vaccine Guide

The Vaccine Guide

Making an
Informed Choice

Randall Neustaedter OMD, LAc.

North Atlantic Books
Homeopathic Educational Services
Berkeley, California

Published by

North Atlantic Books		Homeopathic Educational Services
P.O. Box 12327	and	2124 Kittredge Street
Berkeley, California 94712		Berkeley, California 94704

Cover, book design and production by Catherine E. Campaigne

Printed in the United States of America

The Vaccine Guide: Making an Informed Choice is sponsored by the Society for the Study of Native Arts and Sciences, a nonprofit educational corporation whose goals are to develop an educational and crosscultural perspective linking various scientific, social, and artistic fields; to nurture a holistic view of arts, sciences, humanities, and healing; and to publish and distribute literature on the relationship of mind, body, and nature.

Library of Congress Cataloging-in-Publication Data

Neustaedter, Randall.
    The vaccine guide : making an informed choice / Randall Neustaedter.
        p. cm.
    Includes bibliographical references and index.
    ISBN 1-55643-215-1
        1. Immunization of children—Popular works.   I. Neustaedter, Randall. The immunization decision.   II. Title.
    RJ240.N474   1996
    614.4'7—dc20   95-48308
                                                                                    CIP

4   5   6   7   8   9   10   /   04   03   02   01   00

A major cause of the Roman Empire's decline, after six centuries of world dominance, was its replacement of stone aqueducts by lead pipes for the transport and supply of drinking water. Roman engineers, the best in the world, turned their fellow citizens into neurological cripples. Today our own "best and brightest," with the best of intentions, achieve the same end through childhood vaccination programs yielding the modern scourges of hyperactivity, learning disabilities, autism, appetite disorders, and impulsive violence.

—Harris L. Coulter, Ph.D.

Vaccine Ingredients:

Thimerosal (mercury disinfectant/preservative)
Aluminum (additive to promote antibody response)
Formaldehyde (disinfectant)
Phenol (disinfectant, dye)
Ethylene glycol (antifreeze)
Benzethonium chloride (antiseptic)
Methylparaben (antifungal, preservative)

Warning

Mercury toxicity can result in brain injury and autoimmune disease. Aluminum is associated with Alzheimer's disease and seizures. Formaldehyde causes cancer. It is a hazardous waste and no longer permitted as an ingredient in building insulation.

This book has been written as an information resource for parents. It is not intended as medical advice. As with any medical procedure, parents should base their decisions about vaccines on careful research. Consultation with professionals, including health care providers and attorneys with expertise in the area of vaccination, will also help parents to identify their individual needs.

Contents

Preface

Most parents are surprised to learn that they have a choice about vaccination. Usually, pediatricians do not give parents any information on the vaccine issue. They just begin giving shots, first at a child's birth and then again at the two-month office visit. Parents may have made conscious choices about natural childbirth, circumcision, and breastfeeding, but never considered vaccines.

Who decided this foregone conclusion for them? Why have we adopted a policy of universal immunization with more and more vaccines? One after another the shots come. At each visit parents sign a form, the drug is injected, and the baby screams. Parents are left out of a process too technical for their understanding, and they must trust that someone who makes these rules has their child's best interests in mind.

It is only in recent years that large numbers of people have begun to question the wisdom of the medical world. People are voicing their own choices in health care. Suspicions have been raised. Perhaps the medical system does not have all the right answers after all.

Even amidst the criticisms of the medical establishment, however, very few assail the venerable institution of vaccines. We have been conditioned and convinced to accept these as a savior of children, a miracle that freed us from deadly infectious disease. That battle cry has been repeated so often that it is ingrained in our culture. Politicians concerned about their ratings in the polls pick up a baby and announce their support for more immunizations. In recent memory, President Ford energetically supported the swine flu vaccine catastrophe. President Carter sponsored an immunization campaign that increased Congress's allocated funding from 7 million to 47 million dollars within the first two years after his election. President Reagan passed the National Childhood Vaccine Injury Act of 1986 to ensure adequate vaccine production. And President Clinton passed the Comprehensive Child Immunization Act of 1993. All this was in the name of quality health care for our nation and protection of our children.

Unfortunately, information about the vaccines is not generally available. Parents feel poorly informed. Like most decisions about health care, the choice of which vaccines to give, the timing of vaccines, and their child's safety rests in the hands of the doctor. His or her decision about vaccine administration is governed by vaccine advisory committees, and the committees rely upon studies conducted by drug manufacturers. Any doctor who defies these recommendations risks a malpractice suit or medical-board legal action. Parents who do not make an informed choice place their child's health in the hands of drug companies with a profit motive and doctors who cannot question the recommendations passed down to them.

Parents have the responsibility to provide the best health care possible for their own children. They must decide whether it is better for their child's health to give the vaccines or not. If parents question the validity or wisdom of administering vaccines to their child, they receive little support in their efforts to make an informed choice.

This book is intended to help parents who question the wholesale policy of mass vaccination and its effect on their child. It has two intended functions. One is to give parents information about the diseases, the vaccines, and their adverse effects. Parents need to know the issues and the controversies surrounding these drugs. The potential adverse effects of vaccines are usually hidden from parents. Medical professionals have often stated that broadcasting adverse effects of vaccines to the public would cause unnecessary concern among parents and hinder the vaccine campaign. Dr. Paul Meier summarized this position quite clearly in a panel discussion on the efficacy of the polio vaccine campaign of the 1950s:

It is hard to convince the public that something is good. Consequently, the best way to push forward a new program is to decide on what you think the best decision is and not question it thereafter, and further, not to raise questions before the public or expose the public to open discussion of the issues (Intensive Immunization Programs, Hearings, 1962).

Similar sentiments were recently published again in a dialogue concerning the release of information from a study that suggested the measles vaccine could cause chronic intestinal disease. The Chief Medical Officer of England's Department of Health wrote, "It would be most unfortunate if the publication of this controversial work led to public anxiety over the safety of measles vaccine" (Calman, 1995). The authors of that study responded, "We reported the measles vaccination study for discussion by the scientific community, not only with many qualifications ... but also with great care not to excite media over-reaction.... We realized that the measles vaccination programme is of great importance to the community and the public health of the nation, but it would have been unethical to suppress this result because its preliminary conclusions were uncomfortable or inconvenient" (Thompson *et al.,* 1995a). I would commend the ethical stance of these authors. Unfortunately, information about vaccine reactions is constantly suppressed because such findings run contrary to policy decisions about vaccination.

The recent passage by Congress of the National Vaccine Injury Compensation Act has required more disclosure about vaccines and encouraged informed consent, but parents still have little information about the vaccines, and suppression of information remains a goal of many pharmacies and pediatrician organizations. For example, when the American Academy of Pediatrics' former president, Dr. Martin Smith, reviewed information brochures for parents prepared by the US Department of Health and Human Services, he recommended that they be simplified. He said, "The length and complexity of the materials ... would confuse many parents and could even needlessly alarm them" (AAP News, 1989).

Parents are hungry for information about the vaccines, especially their adverse effects. They are unwilling to blindly accept the opinions of doctors concerning medical care. This book seeks to provide information which is usually unavailable to parents.

The second goal of the book is to increase parental awareness of the issues involved in the use of vaccines. The book places the decision about vaccines within the context of a health care philosophy. Choosing any medical intervention involves personal alignment with a method and a perspective of healing and medicine. Routinely giving vaccines implies tacit approval of a methodology. This book contrasts the approach of modern technological medicine that manipulates the immune system using vaccines with other systems of healing that advocate supporting the body's immune functions. If parents know that choices are available, then they can consider the issues that underlie the use of vaccines. An awareness of the philosophical issues empowers parents to make choices that coincide with their own beliefs. It also provides support for those parents who choose not to vaccinate according to the recommended schedule.

As a primary health care provider for families, one of my responsibilities is to help parents confront the question of vaccines. During the course of these discussions it became clear that parents needed a concise book written by a health care provider that provided a framework for them to make an informed choice regarding vaccinations. This book first appeared in the form of a pamphlet which discussed each of the diseases and their vaccines. When I first wrote the book, parents had few resources available. Since that time several books discussing various aspects of the vaccine controversy have also been published, written from the consumer perspective. The number of vaccines routinely given to children has increased, and the volume of information about vaccine adverse effects has grown astronomically.

The issues can be confusing and overwhelming to parents. In *The Vaccine Guide* I have simplified the issues without sacrificing the detail that parents need to make an informed choice. I present the ideas and facts here as I do with parents in my office. I state the facts about each disease and vaccine, summarize the information, and present the options regarding individual vaccines as well as my recommendations. Ultimately, each parent must decide what is best for their child based on their philosophy, comfort level, and understanding of the real issues that surround vaccinations. Only then will a parent's choice be based upon intelligent reasoning and not blind faith.

I recommend that parents read at least the first chapter, "Making an Informed Choice," and the Conclusion of this book, to understand the philosophical issues involved in making a choice about vaccination. The other chapters about legal requirements and the individual diseases, can be studied later as parents are confronted with each new vaccine.

One note about terminology is warranted here. Throughout the book I use the terms *vaccinate* and *vaccination* rather than *immunize* and *immunization* following the lead of Moskowitz, who states, "The basis of the vaccination controversy is the belief of many parents that the vaccines do not produce a true *immunity,* but rather act in some other fashion—or, in my view, that they act immunosuppressively" (Moskowitz, 1987).

PART I

Choosing

Making an Informed Choice

The experience of childhood vaccination is not pleasant. Babies scream and develop fevers with the first illness of their lives in reaction to the vaccine. Preschoolers learn to fear the doctor because they are jabbed with needles whenever they go for well-child check-ups. Older children run around the doctor's office refusing to be poked, or cling to their mothers in abject terror awaiting the dreaded needle. Parents are informed that vaccines may damage their child's nervous system. This causes understandable apprehension in everyone.

Parents are convinced that all of this is worthwhile. Or are they? Most have doubts, but little information. They have been told that vaccines are the greatest achievement of modern preventive medicine. The polio epidemic of the 1950s, the March of Dimes, and the eradication of smallpox are historical events of the recent past. We are assured that one more generation of vaccines will eliminate whooping cough, measles, and mumps as threats to our children, just as polio and diphtheria have disappeared into memory. This is a reassuring and convincing argument: Risk a few cases of rare adverse effects to eliminate these serious and life-threatening diseases. But lingering doubts remain.

Parents must accommodate themselves to the vaccines' adverse effects. They must steel themselves against their children's inevitable anxiety about the doctor visit and dread of the shot. They wonder about the publicized cases of vaccine-damaged children. Measles, mumps and chickenpox were simple childhood diseases. Why all the excitement about them now? Parents are upset when their child develops a fever after a shot, though it usually is not serious. Parents are devastated if their child develops polio, seizures, or retardation after a vaccination, but these reactions are relatively uncommon. We are told that this is the price we pay for eliminating these diseases from our population. We are reassured that the incidence of these problems would be higher from the natural diseases if the vaccines were not given routinely.

What is the truth about the vaccine campaign? Isn't someone making a lot of money from these billions of shots? Most parents put these doubts aside and rationalize: My pediatrician would not be influenced by a drug company's desire for profit. Doctors would not recommend these vaccines unless they were convinced of their necessity. I have to leave the decision to the doctor. I just don't know enough to make a judgment about such an important issue.

As a parent you are faced with many decisions soon after your baby is born. Most of these are retractable. You can decide to use cloth diapers after four months of plastic ones. If you say the wrong thing to your child, you can recant. If you decide that giving ice cream to Jennifer for breakfast so she gets at least a little protein is not such a great idea after all, you can change your mind tomorrow. Even medical decisions are usually reversible. The decongestant makes Jesse too groggy; let's try a humidifier tonight. But some medical decisions are momentous. Circumcision, vaccination—these are weighty issues with permanent effects.

Parents have a responsibility to avoid toxic exposure and toxic hazards. Poisoning from household chemicals can be prevented by locking up the cupboards and childproofing hazardous areas of the kitchen. Avoiding chemicals in foods takes extra effort. Parents can shop at health-food stores to sidestep the antibiotics and growth hormones in milk, the pesticides on fruits and vegetables, the preservatives in packaged foods. Some toxic exposure cannot be prevented so easily—pollution, ozone depletion, pesticides used on lawns and trees in public parks and playgrounds. Escaping city life may be the only possible solution for these problems. But the toxicity of vaccines, the injection of virulent neurotoxins and heavy metals into an infant's bloodstream, can be avoided by simply saying *no* to the pediatrician.

You must rely on various advisors to give you their opinions. Family, friends, and health professionals can all be helpful and informative, but you must ultimately take responsibility for the choices. The issues of medical decisions are not out of your reach. Except for emergency situations which require immediate action, you can discover the issues and weigh the pros and cons of a medical decision. Some of these may be obvious and simple, others may be agonizing. Any decision will be easier if you have support and reassurance that you are doing the right thing. Unfortunately, the subject of vaccinations often involves heated emotions and recriminations.

I encourage parents to gather information from professionals with differing views about vaccination. The medical issues are controversial, and you need to be aware of these controversies when making a truly informed decision about your child's health care. Individuals with differing perspectives will examine the same data and arrive at different conclusions. For that reason I have included here reviews of the medical literature for parents to examine themselves. I also recommend that parents obtain and read those materials listed at the end of this book that seem most interesting (see Resources). These publications are generally critical of vaccinations for children. Pediatricians and books on child health care are good alternative sources for pro-vaccination information.

I recommend that parents take a careful look at the vaccine question in general and each vaccine individually before making a decision for their child. In the following sections of this book, I outline a practical approach that should help guide you through the maze of the vaccine question.

Four steps are necessary for parents who want to make an informed decision.

1. Understand the philosophical issues surrounding vaccines.
2. Get information about the vaccines.
3. Decide which vaccines you do or don't want.
4. If you decide to vaccinate, then choose the right time.

Philosophy and Medical Care

Modern (allopathic) medicine is based upon several underlying assumptions. The first is the concept of reduction. The body can be reduced to its parts—the organs, the tissues, and the "systems." This allows for the manipulation of one part—the immune system for example—without any regard for the effect this will have on the integrity of the person as a whole. The second assumption is that diseases are bad and need to be combated. This leads to the concept of chemical warfare conducted against the kingdom of diseases. If some innocent civilians lose their lives as a result of the weapons employed, then that is the unfortunate cost of war. This has certainly been the stated position of leaders in the vaccine campaign. The third assumption is that diseases should be prevented by chemicals. This takes the form of lifelong medication with drugs, for example fluoridation of water systems to supposedly prevent tooth decay, estrogen replacement in post-menopausal women to prevent bone loss, and periodic vaccine administration beginning in infancy to prevent infectious diseases.

It is important for parents to examine their beliefs about these assumptions because the administration of vaccines implies tacit approval of the allopathic medical philosophy. Parents do have a choice about the medical treatment of their children. The United States constitution is based upon the principle of freedom of choice. The widespread belief that vaccination of an entire population is necessary, however, has threatened the basic rights of parents and their ability to legally make an informed decision.

The history of mandatory vaccinations reads like the story of martial law in an occupied country. The freedom to choose is suspended in an all-out effort to eradicate an enemy. This is the mentality of war.

The problem with warfare lies in its basically destructive principles. The casualties are usually heavy. In the vaccine war, the casualties have been devastatingly damaged children with resultant lifelong retardation, seizure disorders, autism, and fatalities directly caused by the vaccines.

The crime and the shame of the vaccine industry and the medical establishment have been the routine and blatant denial of these casualties in public testimony and in daily practice. In their view, the good fight has been staged, and these supposed casualties represent merely the deluded suspicions of parents with a sick child who are all too eager to point at vaccines as the cause of their problems. The Vaccine Injury Act was instituted not because the vaccine industry admitted its culpability in these tragedies, but simply because the drug companies refused to continue production of these substances that resulted in multimillion dollar lawsuits. The government chose to subsidize vaccine production by paying awards out of tax dollars and limiting the amount to an administrative budget. Litigation against drug companies was eliminated, and parents were left seeking recompense from a government bureaucracy. This protection of the drug companies assured continuing profits. Vaccine production was re-established. Parents' claims were deflected and continued to be denied, and no further recourse was left to the victims. The war against disease could continue unabated.

The drug companies' production of vaccines and the government's requirements for their administration has been a very successful partnership. When a consumer evaluates medical pronouncements about drug prescriptions for the entire world's population, one should never lose sight of the fact that drug companies reap the tremendous profits. The same companies that make and sell these drugs fund their research. In fact, research and marketing go hand-in-hand. The next simple step is for the drug companies to assist in legislative efforts to make drug-prescribing mandatory for all citizens. The desire for profits has shaped the law.

The war on disease represents the driving force behind vaccine use. The basic assumptions of our culture fuel the policies adopted for our citizens in the areas of medicine and defense. Waging war provides a simple black-and-white perspective: Identify an enemy and declare war. In medicine the concept of disease provides us with the unwitting, elusive, and destructive enemy. The lowly virus and bacterium become the identified targets, the carriers, the weapons, and the tangible troops of the invading army. The analogy is striking. It has become so integrated into our personal belief systems that it seems ludicrous to question it. Who would call disease an ally?

Yet the analogy upon which allopathic medicine is based has no logical foundation. The body is not a battleground. Hostile enemy forces are not threatening our way of life, and biochemical war is not the only solution to illness. There is another philosophy of medicine, which has been ignored in the assumptions of the allopathic world-view. In our population and in our lifetime a shift in consciousness has already occurred. This awareness encompasses the notion that the body itself has an innate intelligence and healing ability.

In this view, the body needs to be nurtured, not attacked with chemicals. The body does have a fundamental order and integrity. This ordered and harmonious function benefits from life-promoting activities, and suffers under the stressful influence of hostile interventions. A philosophy of healing that respects the natural order inherent within the body and the body's innate healing abilities may provide us with an approach to prevention that avoids chemical warfare. When the organism is seen as a whole, when we view nutritional factors, lifestyle, the body's natural integrity, and their overall effect on healing, then we can view vaccines from a different perspective.

All actions have the ability to influence the inherent order of the organism. The body seeks to maintain a healthy balance or homeostasis. Some actions will promote order and others will disorder the internal balance that the body has created. For example, when a child makes a transition from one environment to another, like going to a new preschool, this has the potential to create disorder. The transition may be interpreted by the child as threatening, and the resulting internal disorder might manifest as a tantrum. The parent can then take actions that reassure the child and re-establish balance and homeostasis. Other actions may have a more disordering effect.

To continue the analogy in the emotional realm, the death of a pet or a family member will provoke a deeper injury and greater imbalance. The emotional reactions of fear and grief may cause symptoms. When managed appropriately, with respect for the child's feelings and emotional maturity, these stresses can result in a stronger, more resilient personality. Similarly, different physical stresses on the system will cause varying degrees of imbalance and disorder. When we view the body as an organism in balance, we see everything that occurs as potentially ordering or disordering. An apparent stress can result in order. A continued stress can upset the balance and a toxic stress can cause damage that throws the body into a tailspin.

Drugs have the potential to cause a significant degree of imbalance because of their inherent toxicity. Vaccines can provoke toxic reactions, and they are also capable of causing these same types of imbalances. They can be just as devastating as other severe shocks to the system. The degree of the imbalance and disorder will depend upon the toxic potential of the vaccine and the susceptibility of the organism. By contrast, when an infectious disease causes stress on the body, a vital healing response is mounted as a defense. Marshaling this response can result in a stronger immune system. Illness can thus be seen as a strengthening process, due to its dynamic effect on the body as opposed to the specific antigen-antibody stimulating mechanism of vaccination.

An acute illness can cause a remission of a chronic disease precisely because the acute illness mobilizes healing forces within the body. For example, a recent report in the British medical journal *Lancet* described two patients with multiple sclerosis who experienced remission of their neurologic symptoms after they contracted chickenpox. Both patients had been severely disabled prior to the chickenpox infection. A year later both were participating in normal activities, and one was jogging. Follow-up after two years and six years in the respective cases revealed no further relapse (Ross, 1991). The principle that a similar acute illness can cure a chronic disease was elucidated during the early nineteenth century by Samuel Hahnemann, the founder of homeopathic medicine. Multiple sclerosis and the chickenpox herpes zoster virus both affect the nerves. Hahnemann showed that such an acute infectious disease often cures a chronic problem. In his *Organon of Medicine,* first published in 1810, he said,

> Two diseases, different in nature but very similar in their manifestations and effects, their respective suffering and symptoms, always and infallibly destroy each other as soon as they meet in the organism.... Smallpox ... has removed and cured a host of ills that have similar symptoms.... When measles meets a disease that is similar to it in its main symptom—the eruption—it will undeniably destroy and cure it (Hahnemann, 1982).

The decision about the use of vaccines involves weighing these considerations and viewing them in the context of an underlying philosophy of health and disease.

Looking at the body as a whole, as an integrated organism, encompasses a philosophy in contrast to the allopathic reduction of the body to a set of parts. Modern technological medicine views only short-term reactions and the localized effects of its interventions. There is little attention paid to long-term effects because there is no model for viewing or evaluating these. The double-blind study looks at limited effects on distinct physiological systems in the body. Vaccines stimulate specific antibody responses in the immune system. That is the desired effect, and the ultimate goal is prevention of a specific disease in the tested population. These tests run for a few years at the most. The issue of long-term detrimental effects of vaccines never arises in these study designs because that concept defies the nature of those tests.

Politically, it would not be useful to look for these effects because the studies are conducted by vaccine manufacturers and the government, both of whom have a vested interest in the product and a long-term political and monetary commitment to the promotion of the vaccine campaign. They have no interest in revealing vaccine toxicity. This intentionally myopic view encourages the limited perspective of allopathic medicine, but parents and consumers of medical services are questioning this limited view. They increasingly seek the perspectives of other medical systems that do view the body as a whole.

The systems of Traditional Chinese Medicine (TCM), homeopathy, naturopathy, and Ayurvedic medicine all share the belief that interventions have global, long-term effects in the body. The goal of these systems is to bring the body into a higher state of order and balance. Their interventions create harmony. Within these systems, diet, drug use, herbs, medicines, exercise, emotions, thoughts, beliefs, and relationships all play a role in the overall health of each person. The physical body and the mind are linked in the sense that an imbalance in one realm will affect other realms. Physical illness can cause emotional stress, and emotional turmoil can cause physical reactions. When the natural energetic balance and harmony of body systems is upset, then the resulting disorder may manifest in symptoms and destructive physiological processes. A persistent unremitting stress may cause chronic problems. For example, repressed anger can result in physical changes within the body, causing high blood pressure or a depressed immune system and consequent cancer growth.

Vaccine critics have postulated that the constant stress caused by manipulating and altering the immune system with vaccines could also result in these types of imbalances and disease processes. Healing systems that address these imbalances intend the opposite effect— to create harmony and re-establish balance in the body. The goal is a healthy life and prevention of illness. The crisis-oriented approach of allopathic medicine and its attention to isolated, disjointed reactions exists in sharp distinction to the curative and preventive healing approaches of these other medical systems.

A shift has occurred in the West, from a fear of isolated diseases towards a focus on the organism as a whole and the strength of its immune response. Fear of disease has fueled the fire of allopathic medicine throughout its history and caused a preoccupation with infection. Perhaps this was appropriate during medieval and early industrial historical periods, when infectious disease ran rampant. In the era of waste-disposal technology systems, the frequency and severity of these diseases has steadily declined. Perhaps shifting the focus away from fear and the toxic weapons of war (antibiotics and vaccines) is now appropriate for our culture.

The subject of immune system deficiencies has occupied a great deal of attention in the health care industry, especially the health-foods arena. Many products now exist that purport to strengthen the immune system including herbs, mushrooms, and algae, as well as meditation, and movement techniques. This interest stems from the widespread rise in immune system disorders and in new diseases that never existed prior to the modern chemical era of industrial pollution and drugs (AIDS, cancer, lupus, chronic fatigue syndrome, hypothyroidism, and a whole array of autoimmune disorders). Opportunistic viruses may also play a role in the declining health of the population, but concern over the fundamental underlying immune system failure lies at the core of the efforts to develop immune enhancement.

The possible role of vaccines in causing these immune system deficiencies has been the subject of much speculation and controversy. Many health care providers and consumer advocates have pointed to vaccines as a cause of immune failure. The coincident emergence of these diseases and the mass vaccination of populations has led to suspicions that an entire generation has suffered immune system crippling from the vaccines that should be protecting us from illness. Eloquent indictments about the toxic effects of vaccines on immune system function have recently been written, and parents would do well to consider the information they contain (Scheibner, 1993; Murphy, 1993; Miller, 1992). Other body systems may also be impacted by the vaccines. The nervous system seems to be particularly sensitive to the toxic properties of vaccines. Subtle nervous system damage caused by vaccines has been identified as a possible source of the recently identified epidemic problems of attention disorders, criminal behavior in children, and the emergence of autism as a new disease since the advent of mass vaccination (Coulter, 1990). More immediate and dramatic nervous system reactions can occur soon after vaccine administration, often after the third or fourth dose. These include convulsions sometimes resulting in lifelong epilepsy, persistent high-pitched screaming, bizarre grimacing, and sudden unexplainable death (SIDS). Of course, these types of reactions are continuously denied by the vaccine industry (Institute of Medicine, 1994).

Another significant shift in consciousness that affects the way parents make health care decisions includes the evolving view of the doctor. Some parents have discovered that the exalted position of the medical doctor who dictates all treatment decisions may involve misplaced trust. Doctors are trained by drug companies, both in medical schools and later in their offices and clinics. Medical textbooks teach drug prescribing, clinical training involves learning the proper way to prescribe drugs, and seminars for doctors in practice teach the latest advances in drug development. All of this information is derived from research conducted by the pharmaceutical industry, whose only goal is to sell drugs. Increasingly, drug companies own the health care delivery institutions themselves. In this way they can supervise and design the delivery of their products.

This phenomenon has not escaped the consumer's awareness. If an individual citizen in the role of patient wants something other than drugs, then he or she must turn to sources outside the medical establishment simply because the world of physicians represents the position of the drug-manufacturing industry. Many parents have realized that accepting the opinion of their physician about vaccines is similar to believing the car salesman's pitch. Both have a product to push. Vaccines represent consumer goods—and parents should research this product far more carefully than other purchases because their children's lives could be at stake.

The doctor-as-God philosophy is gradually losing ground. Consumers want information. The scandals and tragedies associated with drug company products have created a more wary public. Thalidomide, the IUD, silicone breast implants, and unnecessary mutilations in the form of mastectomies and hysterectomies have resulted in widespread mistrust. People have discovered that drug companies may not have our best interests at heart. Doctors do what they are told. The consumer who does not beware is the unwitting participant and potential victim.

A Personal Choice

What constitutes personal choice in health care decisions? The first parameter involves the freedom to choose. When some group or authority dictates policies, there can be no personal decision. This freedom is a fundamental right, and yet parents in many states have been denied the right to choose whether their children are injected with chemicals recommended by the vaccine industry. The requirement to vaccinate makes parents criminals if they refuse to comply. Religious and medical exemptions to vaccination merely place the decision in the hands of another authority, the church or the doctor. This well-guarded authority has been upheld by courts in some states, which require that parents prove their membership in a recognized church that proscribes vaccines before they qualify for a religious exemption. If parents who live in those states do make a personal decision that a particular vaccine is too toxic for their child, they cannot exercise their right to choose avoidance of vaccines. The remaining states that do provide parents with the option of a personal belief or philosophical exemption to vaccination at least allow parents to choose for themselves.

The second parameter in a personal decision requires that you assess your own needs. This involves getting information, weighing your choices, and evaluating the pros and cons of an issue. The reasoning for a family may differ from the reasoning for an entire population. You may find that your needs are significantly different than those of someone else. For example, is your child at a higher risk than the general population due to overcrowding, poor nutrition, and inadequate sanitation? These are factors that could make an individual child more susceptible and more likely to come in contact with infectious diseases.

A public health official may have a completely different agenda for the nation than you do for your own family. The strategy for eliminating diseases from a population usually includes universal measures for everyone, regardless of risk of exposure or consequences for the individual. The population takes precedence over the individual. The following quote taken from an article in the British medical journal, *Lancet,* makes this abundantly clear.

> There is still much to be learned about how best to use vaccines for maximum benefit to the community as well as to the individual. For a pathogenic microbe to persist within a population, the density of susceptible individuals needs to exceed a critical value such that, on average, each primary case of infection generates at least one secondary. Thus, it may be to the benefit of society as a whole for an individual to be immunised but in that individual's interest not to be! As with other matters bearing on altruism in society, the promotion of vaccination to secure herd immunity raises complex issues (Moxon, 1990).

The "complex issue" to an epidemiologist amounts to this for an individual parent: Are you willing to sacrifice your child to satisfy a public health official's objectives? Some children will inevitably be sacrificed to achieve certain goals for the community. Are you prepared to take that risk with your child? In answering that question, consider whether you agree with the philosophy that underlies the methods. Is it necessary or even wise to wipe out diseases, to prevent the body's management of childhood illnesses, to manipulate the immune system, beginning at birth, with toxic chemicals? What is the risk from these diseases? What are the dangers of vaccines? Why have parents not been told about the devastating reactions that can occur? This massive marketing scheme has been heralded as the greatest preventive health measure of modern times, brought to us by the pharmaceutical industry and their vaccine researchers. It is time that vaccines and their promotion campaign be viewed with a critical eye. Are you ready to inject these powerful and toxic drugs into your child, on the advice of drug manufacturers, at the insistence of doctors who are paid by these drug companies, delivered to you by doctors trained by those same companies? Look at the facts, and reach your own conclusions.

Organizations of parents have been formed to fight the policy of mandatory vaccines for children. These parents represent their vaccine-injured children. They have learned about vaccines because their toxic effects destroyed their child's health. Listen to their experience and see their side before you meekly rest assured in the word of your doctor, who tells you exactly what he was told by the drug company. Question the effects of drugs used on your child. These are not difficult issues to understand. You can take control of these decisions. Make sure that you feel comfortable in your choices. Do not become the naive victim of wholesale drug policies. This is an area of your life and your family's health that you can control.

Let's consider an example of how drug-company recommendations can influence your pediatrician and government policy about vaccines. The following facts represent just one drama in the vaccine world, where billions of dollars in revenues and vaccine-injury claims are at stake. In 1990, Marie Griffin and her associates at Vanderbilt University School of Medicine in Nashville, Tennessee published a study on the risk of seizures and other neurologic events following the DTP (Diphtheria-Tetanus-Pertussis) vaccine. This study appeared in the *Journal of the American Medical Association (JAMA)*. The study was big in scope, including more than 38,000 children who received 107,000 doses of DTP. Their conclusion? "No child who was previously normal without a prior history of seizures had a seizure in the 0 to 3 days following vaccination that marked the onset of either epilepsy or other neurological or developmental abnormality." This seems to provide the final word about the supposed neurotoxicity of the pertussis vaccine and brain damage (encephalopathy). Accompanying the article, an editorial titled, " 'Pertussis vaccine encephalopathy': It is time to recognize it as the myth that it is," by James Cherry, proclaimed the end of the long debate about pertussis vaccine and nervous system damage. He said,

It is now the last decade of the 20th century, and it is time for the myth of pertussis vaccine encephalopathy to end.... Unfortunately, because of the sensationalistic media, the organization of a group of parents who attribute their children's illnesses and deaths to pertussis vaccine, and the unique destructive force of personal-injury lawyers, we now have a national problem that shouldn't be.... We need to end this national nonsense. To do this, we need vaccine information relating to risks and benefits that represent true scientific evidence (such as reviewed in this report) and not the wishes of special interest groups (Cherry, 1990).

Later that year, Vincent Fulginiti published another editorial titled, "A pertussis vaccine myth dies," in another AMA sponsored journal, *The American Journal of Diseases of Children (AJDC)*. He cites the study and Dr. Cherry, relating his own spin on the controversy:

Many years ago, I believed, as did most vaccine investigators at the time, that a certain number of children were permanently damaged by the toxic influence of pertussis vaccine on the brain. We held this belief because of published anecdotal reports, added to our own limited individual experience as infectious disease consultants, of patients who experienced neurologic disorders in temporal association with receipt of pertussis vaccine.... Why do parents and some physicians persist in their fervent belief that pertussis vaccine causes permanent neurologic damage? ... Some parents believe that personal tragedy must have some retribution. If the vaccine caused it, then the doctor or the manufacturer should pay. I suspect that some individuals pursue lawsuits out of greed, but most do so because it assuages their conscience, i.e., it brings "justice" into a tragic clinical circumstance (Fulginiti, 1990).

Similar editorials occurred across the nation (California Department of Health Services, 1994). Several problems, however, taint the purity of these clinical studies and their interpretation. First, Marie Griffin was reported to be

financially supported by Burroughs Wellcome, one of the world's largest pertussis (whooping cough) vaccine manufacturers. Griffin, Burroughs-Wellcome Scholar in Pharmacology at Vanderbilt University, was the principal author. . . . As a result of Griffin's study JAMA published an editorial calling for an end to the federal vaccine injury compensation system on the grounds that the pertussis vaccine does not cause permanent brain damage. . . . James Cherry, MD, of UCLA, is a paid consultant for Lederle Laboratories, the largest American manufacturer of pertussis vaccine (Conflict . . . , 1990).

Fulginiti, as editor of AJDC, chose to publish a disclaimer about his drug-company affiliations.

Many years ago he received support from a variety of pharmaceutical firms to undertake studies of many vaccines, including pertussis vaccine. He has also, in the past but not in recent years, testified as an expert witness for physicians and pharmaceutical firms, for which he received compensation, in trials concerning the alleged side effects of pertussis vaccine (Fulginiti, 1990).

This situation of vaccine researchers simultaneously working for the pharmaceutical industry and also evaluating the studies for physician groups is such a common practice that no one questions the conflict of interest involved in this closed loop. Cherry was paid by the vaccine-production companies and also headed the 1988 American Academy of Pediatrics task force on pertussis and pertussis immunization, whose report also denied any major problems with the vaccine. In their dismissal of a British study that did show a significant association between the vaccine and serious neurologic disorders, they concluded, "The data can be interpreted as demonstrating a temporal association in which DTP calls attention to or brings out something that is to occur anyway but is just moved forward in time because of the immunization" (Cherry *et al.*, 1988). The drug manufacturers blame the parents for seeking retribution against them, and claim that vaccine-injured children would have acquired these problems anyway. Then the government steps in to protect the drug companies. Who is in control here?

All of the denial and self-congratulation in this particular drama were based on the findings of the Griffin study. But the quality and methods of that study itself were called into question. For example, the identified cases included only those vaccine recipients who

experienced a "first nonneonatal seizure or episode of encephalopathy that resulted in Medicaid reimbursement for a medical encounter
between the first DTP immunization and the end of study follow-
up." Coulter, in his critique of this study, asks, "How about the children who did not apply for a Medicaid reimbursement? Not every
parent rushes to the Medicaid office for medicines just because the
child has seizures or 'spells'" (Coulter, 1990a). He goes on to criti-
cize the research methods.

> The authors found 1187 cases which matched their case
> definition, but then proceeded to exclude most of them with-
> out providing the reader with adequate justification for so
> doing. Thus (p. 1643), 359 were excluded because their records
> were "not available for review." Why did the authors of the
> study not go out to the homes of these children and get the
> records or interview the parents? . . . This is especially regret-
> table, even reprehensible, as the authors admit that about
> half of them (147 cases) seemed to meet their case definition.
> They had "non hospital based outpatient records only, which
> were not available to us." If they can't get the materials, they
> shouldn't publish the study.

The study also looked at deaths following the vaccine. They found
that in a period of 15 to 30 days after vaccination, there was a 20
percent increase in deaths compared to the control group. Yet in their
summary they say only that they found no increased risk of SIDS in
the 0-to-14-day interval after DTP vaccination. This exclusion of possible late effects allows them to "conclude that in this large population of children there was no increase in the risk of SIDS after
immunization with the DTP vaccine" (Coulter, 1990b). In reviewing
the "Results" section of that study, Coulter remarks, "This section I
find almost impossible to understand, full of gratuitous assumptions,
overlapping categories, and the like. Actually, considering the method-
ological errors made already in designing and carrying out the study,
the results don't mean much." In reference to the "Conclusions" section, which says, in part, "serious neurological events are rarely, if
ever, caused by DTP immunization," Coulter notes, "These are tor-
tured sentences that seem clearly designed to conceal some nasty
findings but to allow the authors an escape route if anyone calls them
on this study" (Coulter, 1990a).

Similarly, in a discussion of Cherry's editorial dismissing the supposed myth of pertussis encephalopathy, another reviewer also criticized the methods and conclusions of the Griffin study.

> The studies endorsed by Cherry as proving no permanent brain damage from pertussis toxin have never operationally defined comprehensively or examined with reliable detection measures the full range of pertussis toxin-produced encephalopathies. Neither office neurological examinations nor Medicaid mothers' reporting of frank or partial complex seizures is a reliable system of measurement for detecting mild to moderate pertussis vaccine encephalopathies.... (Lewis, 1990).

Since the Griffin article appeared and the vaccine industry so readily dismissed any association between the pertussis vaccine and neurologic sequelae, other studies have continued to reveal the vaccine's problems. Apparently, other researchers did not believe that the "myth" had been put to rest. A follow-up survey was conducted of the children identified as suffering "severe acute neurological events within seven days of pertussis immunisation" in the famous British study conducted ten years prior. This survey showed that after ten years, "significantly more children with such illnesses die or suffer subsequent educational, behavioural, or neurological deficits than expected by comparison with controls" (Miller et al., 1993).

Another study published the same year as the Griffin study also showed a positive association between severe acute neurologic illnesses and recent administration of DTP vaccine (Gale *et al.*, 1990). Either these studies have continued to perpetuate the "myth" of vaccine damage to the nervous system, or the vaccine defenders were suspiciously premature in their verdicts. A summary of the evidence, including the Griffin article, published by the American Academy of Pediatrics, seemed to agree. The authors conclude with two points: "1. There is an association between DTP vaccine and serious acute neurologic illness.... 2. We do not know whether pertussis vaccine causes permanent brain damage" (Wentz & Marcuse, 1991). Nonetheless, the vaccine defenders made their point, which was echoed in the popular press. The drama merely reflects the high stakes involved in the form of salaries, profits, and the defense of a personal belief.

Anyone who doubts the culpability of the vaccine industry in suppressing information, distorting research, and manipulating the public would do well to read the sobering account of this corruption in the book *A Shot in the Dark*. There we learn, for example, that in 1988 James Cherry admitted receiving $50,000 per year for testifying in lawsuits on behalf of vaccine manufacturers in vaccine damage-cases, obtained $400,000 in grant funds for UCLA, partly covering his expenses and salary, and that his department at UCLA received $450,000 in "gifts" from Lederle Laboratories.

With such powerful combined forces at work—the vaccine manufacturers, medical associations, government committees, legislature, and media—it is not surprising that vaccine acceptance pervades our culture. Public health policies support this vast industry. Considering the range of organizations and forces involved in this field, a multitude of motives emerges that drive the vaccine campaign.

First and foremost is modern medicine. The medical world has very little to offer in the treatment of infectious disease. This impotence in the face of illness leads to a strong desire to prevent these untreatable problems, even at a high cost in the form of adverse effects. Viruses and whooping cough are not responsive to antibiotics. That covers measles, mumps, rubella, polio, chickenpox, hepatitis, and pertussis. But more and more bacteria have become resistant to antibiotics. That threatens the effectiveness of the few drugs that treat the remaining microbes in question, *Haemophilus,* diphtheria, and tetanus.

The ineffectiveness of allopathic medicine creates a compelling desire to develop vaccines, which shifts the research arm of the industry into hyperdrive. The fact that other forms of treatment could be utilized to treat the infectious diseases is ignored. Allopathic medicine denies the effectiveness of any treatment besides its own drugs. The model does not allow for recognition of other healing systems. This occurs even when another healing modality proves effective. Generally, this merely encourages the harshness of the medical world's opposition. For example, when homeopathic medicine proved clinically effective in treating yellow-fever epidemics and severe influenza outbreaks, the allopathic medical establishment redoubled its efforts to discredit and destroy the competition (Coulter, 1973). Modern medicine has bet its money on vaccines to such an extent that the belief in their goodness pervades all discussions. The universally accepted credo that the benefits derived from vaccines outweigh their risks fuels the research, adoption, and dissemination of vaccines despite any evidence that they may be harmful.

The nearly compulsive desire to wipe out diseases governs public health policies. In this great battle we lose lives to vaccine injuries. Even this unfortunate fact is vehemently denied. The obvious self-justification that more lives would be lost to the disease is a specious and convenient argument that ends discussion. The medical world first blinds itself to the possibility of treating these illnesses with anything beyond its own meager methods, then justifies its use of toxic drugs to wipe out the offenders. The concept of mutual existence between humans and these microbes has never been considered. The possibility that the body can be encouraged to manage these diseases has never entered the worldview of modern medicine. This results in a simple, self-perpetuating philosophy: Vaccines are good, diseases are bad. And this war cry is echoed throughout the modern world.

The vaccine business also provides jobs for physicians. Positions for vaccine experts occur in the form of pharmaceutical researchers, academic researchers, and membership on professional organization and government committees. This medical wing of the vaccine industry supports itself through promotion of vaccines. Their promotion of vaccines ensures self-employment, continuation of research funds, and academic positions.

Drug manufacturers realized that the allopathic goal of wiping out diseases held the promise of vast fortunes. They were quick to combine forces and supply physicians with the armaments for their massive campaign. Vaccine researchers have provided the vaccine manufacturers with a guaranteed world market for their product. Their alliance in this effort is apparent at all public hearings, government committee meetings, and court cases involving vaccine toxicity and injuries to children. The vaccine producers have one goal—profits. They will produce a vaccine for anything if they are guaranteed a market, especially if they are protected from lawsuits. They are not motivated by improving world health. They are not willing to lose money on vaccines. If vaccines stop producing a profit, they stop producing vaccines, a simple equation.

Government provides the seal of approval for the vaccine campaign. Politicians get into the vaccine business because of their own personal beliefs, their alliance with the medical establishment viewpoint, and their need to adopt popular causes. Protecting children and improving the health status of disadvantaged populations represent noncontroversial political positions. If the pharmaceutical industry profits from such government decisions, so much the better. They mount a tremendous lobbying effort, and mandatory vaccine policies translate to lucrative gold-mines. Testifying at government hearings, providing expert paid researchers for government committees, advising politicians about vaccine campaign plans—all represent solid marketing strategies. After all, the government is a vaccine company's biggest single customer. There is no mystery in the motives of vaccine manufacturers' efforts to sponsor and lobby for state legislation that requires vaccination for school entry. Every new vaccine's marketing strategy includes vast sums from the manufacturer, SmithKline, Merck, or Lederle, to get it mandated for the entire population of children in every state.

For many reasons, the factors that influence a government to adopt vaccine requirements may differ considerably from the individual parent's personal goals for a family. Politicians, vaccine companies, and medical organizations have their own concerted agenda for their immunization campaign. This agenda may coincide with your choices as a consumer of medical services, or it may not. Since administering the vaccines involves significant health risks for your child, it makes sense to base your choice on health considerations for the individual and not on a public policy determined by drug companies.

Vaccine promoters make the claim that everyone must continue to comply with government recommendations or the diseases will return; but they have no proof that this will occur. The much-touted success of vaccine campaigns is debatable in any case. The incidence of the diseases in question has consistently declined over the past hundred years. Vaccines in current use have only been widely used since the 1940s, and some are much more recent. The pressure to vaccinate is founded upon vaccine company claims, and a commitment to a belief system that runs deeply in economic and philosophical veins. Parents should be aware of the motives and methods involved in these public health measures.

When it comes to making a choice about whether or not to vaccinate, parents usually have two simultaneous voices vying for their attention. If they have come this far in their thinking, if they are questioning whether it is actually wise to give their child these shots, then doubts have crept into the equation. They are not absolutely sure that the pediatrician is telling them the whole story. They are not altogether convinced. The doubts speak through an instinctual, protective, parental voice. They have heard about adverse vaccine effects through friends, or articles and books. They want information, but their pediatrician is not forthcoming. All they get from that side is calm reassurance that the vaccines are safe, that the diseases represent a far greater risk. It is a comforting paternalistic tone that lulls their distracting doubts and intimidates them through a subtle coercion. Belief systems cannot really be questioned; too much time is usually spent attempting to prove that they are correct.

Some parents, however, continue to question the accepted wisdom despite the heresy this entails. They want to be responsible and make the right decision. An internal voice says, maybe giving all these vaccines is not the best thing to do right now. My baby seems so vulnerable and delicate. Maybe we could wait.

Confronted with this, the pediatrician usually becomes furious and accusatory. Parents remain in a quandary. If they have little information, they usually succumb. With no support for their doubts, they capitulate. Only the most stalwart parents continue to pursue their questions. In most cases, the second voice raises its competing song. This voice doubts the doubting voice. How could all of these people be wrong about vaccines? We must be crazy to question what is so accepted by everyone around us. Lulled thus into submission, the first voice often turns tail and slips off gain. It returns fleetingly when the mother watches the syringe enter her baby's skin, sees her baby scream, and dreads the possible reactions she has acknowledged when signing off her informed consent.

Anxiety is the keynote of this internal fugue. Emotions run high when confronting time-honored beliefs. Ultimately, a parent's choice comes down to one question: Are we more anxious about the diseases or the vaccines? The fear of diseases runs deep in our culture. Anxiety on this score already tops the charts. It is fueled by vivid stories recounting the horrors of infectious diseases of bygone eras, deaths from diphtheria, and iron-lung hospital wards during the great polio wars. High drama in the fight against disease provides the backdrop for the savior legends of modern medicine, glorifying the inventors of vaccines, Pasteur, Salk, and Sabin. Anxiety about diseases stirs easily in the parental breast.

Anxiety about vaccines runs along more nebulous lines. Parents have few resources to inform them about problems with vaccines. Their fear of vaccines stems from their own childhood experiences with needles. They have personally felt the initial pain and the subsequent illness caused by vaccines. Inflicting this on their children is not a pleasant prospect. Of course, this anxiety is consciously repressed because of its illogical nature.

Other anxieties stem from hearsay and second-hand information that sporadically leaks into mainstream culture. Reports of the dangers associated with vaccines are vehemently denied by the vast industry that controls the media. In 1982, when NBC-TV released a vaccine exposé that revealed the devastating damage to children caused by the pertussis vaccine, the Centers for Disease Control (CDC), the American Medical Association (AMA), and the American Association of Pediatrics (AAP) called it biased, histrionic, amoral, and psychopathic. The producer of the show said the American press did not pick up the story "because doctors have squelched it" (Coulter, 1991). Parents have little access to these reports unless they subscribe to magazines such as *Mothering* that continually recount the problems associated with vaccines.

There is little support for parent's doubts. Their anxieties are labeled hysterical, and then repudiated. Parents wonder if their concerns are exaggerated. Given their doubts about vaccine safety and the doubts about these doubts, it is no wonder that parents are confused. In fact, parents have anxiety about vaccines because they sense and know the physical stress on the system that vaccines do cause. They have experienced this in their own bodies, and in the reactions of their children. In some children this reaction presents more obvious symptoms than in others. Parents who have seen dramatic changes in their child's behavior following a vaccine will be more anxious about the next one in the schedule. If their children make it through the vaccine reaction without developing severe symptoms, then they breathe a sigh of relief and think, "there, it wasn't so bad after all."

Going against the grain, rejecting an almost universally held belief that vaccines have saved us from disease and refusing them, causes painful experiences for parents. Self-doubt creeps in and parents wonder, have I done the right thing? Grandparents, friends and medical providers become accusatory. Standing firm in the choice can be difficult. Parents often need support and continual reinforcement that they have made the right choice. Overcoming the anxiety instilled by such deep cultural expectations may require time, patience, and repeated exposure to views that question the authoritative statements of the vaccine industry that continually bombard parents.

One thing that vaccines surely accomplish is the relief of parental guilt. When parents consent to the vaccines, they rest assured in the belief that they have done everything humanly possible in modern medicine. If the disease strikes, then it was an unfortunate case of vaccine failure, a not uncommon event. (Ninety percent or more of measles cases in some epidemics occur in those previously vaccinated.) If a crippling reaction to a vaccine occurs, at least parents do not feel guilty, because they did what they were told. They may be angry and distraught, but they reassure themselves that it was not their fault; they did what they were told. The less thinking that occurs prior to giving the vaccine, the less guilt. This places all the authority and all the responsibility on the shoulders of vaccine experts who dictate the path that parents must follow. If their motives are not always in the best interest of the individual child, well, parents will never discover it.

Options: Choosing and Timing Vaccines

What options are available to parents in their choice about vaccines? First, parents may decide they want less than the total range of recommended vaccines. It comes as a surprise to some parents that they can choose to have one or some vaccines and refuse others. You are responsible for your child's health. You are in control. If a child suffers a dramatic and tragic reaction to a vaccine, it is the parents who must cope with it. The doctors may be sympathetic, but they are personally uninvolved. They view it merely as a casualty in the war against disease, if they admit any culpability at all.

When would a parent choose to give some vaccines and not others? Simply stated, some vaccines apparently represent a more dangerous threat to the body than others. This is inferred from the types of immediate, short-term reactions that we can observe. We assume that those vaccines with the most dramatic short-term toxicity also pose a more dangerous risk for long-term reactions, though this has not been proven because no one has studied the long-term effects of vaccines.

Given that the long-term risks are unknown, parents usually make choices about individual vaccines based on the history of short-term reactions they have caused. The pertussis, measles, and rubella vaccines tend to cause more significant observable reactions than others, though hepatitis and polio vaccines can also cause serious illness. The most commonly avoided vaccine is pertussis because by now, after more than sixty years of medical reports of horrific reactions (deaths, epilepsy, and retardation) from the whole-cell pertussis vaccine, public fear of the vaccine has mounted. The fact that many other countries have abandoned the pertussis vaccine has strengthened the resolve of many parents to also refuse the vaccine. These parents have held their ground, and many physicians, though they may not take the same position, admit that a parent's concern about possible reactions may be justified, despite the consistent denial of the American vaccine industry.

Parents can pick and choose from the list of vaccines based on their own individual family's needs and their own research. They may decide that some diseases pose enough danger to their child to risk the adverse effects of the vaccine. Even a parent who has rejected most vaccines because of their potential adverse effects may choose to give one or a few individual vaccines. Typically, tetanus is a disease that concerns many parents. Since the vaccine causes less immediate severe reactions than others, because the vaccine always works to prevent tetanus, and because tetanus represents a life-threatening situation when it does occur, parents who refuse other vaccines sometimes opt to get the tetanus shots for their child. A parent's concern may be greater for a very active child, especially around horses, since both these factors increase the risk of wounds and exposure to tetanus. Other families may be considering travel to areas of the world (Asia or Africa) where polio still exists, and they will consider giving that vaccine even if they realize that polio does not occur in their own part of the world.

Typically, parents will avoid and refuse specific vaccines for two reasons. Either they fear serious vaccine reactions because of a vaccine's history, or the disease causes so little concern that the vaccine does not seem necessary to them. These vaccines are listed in Table 1. Other diseases represent a greater threat, and parents may feel more secure giving the vaccine than risking the disease in their child.

Table 1

Vaccines That Parents Commonly Refuse

High vaccine toxicity	*Low disease incidence or severity*
Pertussis	Chickenpox
Acellular pertussis	Hepatitis
Measles	Diphtheria
Mumps	Polio
Rubella	

Table 2

Diseases That Commonly Concern Parents the Most

Tetanus

Haemophilus

Polio

Diphtheria

The most difficult aspect of rejecting or refusing vaccines may be finding a cooperative pediatrician or family physician. The decision itself can be complicated and agonizing. Parents must consider conflicting opinions and resources, including unsolicited advice, and then search their own hearts and minds for the answers that make sense to them. Through this process their child also may require a medical provider as a resource for health problems, concerns, or for general advice. It may be difficult to find a compassionate and understanding doctor who will respect and accept parents' decisions about vaccine use for their child. When interviewing a potential doctor, the question of his or her position about the issue of parental choice concerning vaccines may be crucial to their search.

Increasingly, parents may not have a choice about their child's doctor. They must take what they get from their health care plan. Parents may need to steel themselves for a fight. The pressure exerted by doctors to give vaccines is enormous. Many pediatricians in private practice will refuse to care for children whose parents refuse vaccines. Doctors will often bully and harass parents who question them or who refuse vaccines for their child. It takes a strong parent to confront this kind of blatant persecution.

Since the medical establishment's certainty about vaccines constitutes a belief system, any other view is considered heresy. The more zealous defenders of vaccine policies and promoters of the mass vaccine campaign will sometimes vehemently confront parents, and have even proposed seeking out these recalcitrant citizens. Parents should be on their guard when discussing vaccines with medical professionals, schools, or government administrators. Doctors have accused parents of neglect and even contacted Child Protective Services upon discovering that a child was not fully vaccinated. So far, federal legislation that proposed tracking children's vaccine status in a computerized database has failed to be enacted due to the efforts of parent advocacy groups. This would allow state governments to seek and find families who refuse vaccines.

An understanding doctor will provide support and comfort to families who confront the *status quo* of vaccine laws. A caring family doctor or pediatrician should respect parents enough to accept their well-considered decisions about vaccine use for their own family. He or she may even be willing to write a medical exemption for admittance to schools.

The second option that parents can consider concerns the timing of vaccines. It is not necessary to begin giving vaccines at birth or two months of age. Delaying vaccines will at least give you time to make your choices. It will also give your baby's body a chance to develop a less vulnerable immune system and nervous system, which are so susceptible to the vaccines' toxic effects. Delay of DTP vaccination until two years of age in Japan resulted in a dramatic decrease in adverse vaccine effects. During the period 1970 through 1974, when DTP vaccine was begun at 3 to 5 months of age, the Japanese national compensation system paid claims for 57 permanent severe vaccine reactions and 37 deaths. During the following six-year period, 1975 through 1980, when DTP vaccine was begun at 24 months of age, severe reactions were reduced to a total of eight with three deaths (Noble *et al.*, 1987). This is an 85 to 90 percent reduction in severe reactions and deaths calculated according to total doses of vaccine administered during these years. Dr. James Cherry and colleagues, reporting the American Academy of Pediatrics Task Force on Pertussis findings, conclude, "It is clear that delaying the initial vaccination until a child is 24 months ... reduces most of the temporally associated severe adverse events" (Cherry *et al.*, 1988).

Delaying the initiation of vaccines in a child will not reduce the effectiveness of the vaccine. In fact, the early administration of vaccines has created problems with effective antibody production in response to the vaccine itself. For example, measles, mumps and rubella vaccines do not produce persistent antibody responses if they are administered prior to 15 months of age. The effort to manufacture more effective vaccines has focused on the issue of how soon a vaccine can be used and still maintain persistent effects over time. So if you delay giving vaccines to your child, then the length of effectiveness will probably be enhanced.

Only two diseases that have corresponding vaccines cause any significant problems within the first year of life in countries with modern sanitation systems. These two are whooping cough (pertussis) and *Haemophilus* meningitis. The pertussis vaccine has caused so many dangerous reactions that Western European countries consider its use unjustifiable and have eliminated it from the roster of routinely administered vaccines. If you decide not to give the pertussis vaccine for the same reasons, then the remaining vaccine to consider is *Haemophilus*. This is a relatively new and experimental vaccine, only licensed for use in infants since 1990. The risk of exposure to *Haemophilus* for infants under one year increases in large day care settings, so this may be a consideration for you. Parents should carefully read the discussion in the *Haemophilus* chapter.

Certain other diseases—diphtheria, tetanus, polio, hepatitis, and chickenpox—do not threaten babies. Diphtheria and polio do not exist in the United States. The possibility of exposure to tetanus is extremely unlikely in a child under two years old, since tetanus can only be acquired from an injury to the skin such as a puncture wound. Hepatitis is primarily a sexually transmitted disease, and chickenpox causes minimal problems if acquired during childhood at any age. Delaying vaccination causes minimal risk of disease and can result in a dramatically reduced risk of toxic reactions. After infancy your child has developed his or her own antibody production mechanisms and a more resilient defense system for coping with toxic substances. Even if you do nothing else outside the recommended or state-required vaccine onslaught on the body, you might consider the delay of this attack on the system until your child is beyond infancy and less vulnerable to vaccine reactions.

Vaccines are usually recommended for use during infancy, as opposed to some later age, for two reasons. First, the incidence of diseases that do pose a health risk to infants can be reduced in this way. This assumes that the individual vaccine is effective, which may or may not be true.

The second, and much more important, reason is that doctors have access to babies during the first year of life. Parents dutifully bring their babies for well-child check-ups every two or three months during infancy. This provides the perfect opportunity to give several doses of vaccines. The recommended vaccine schedule has been devised to conform to this spacing of check-ups. After two years of age, children would not normally visit their doctor every few months for any reason other than shots if the vaccines were begun at that age.

The timing of this medical intervention has evolved out of convenience and the strategies of a mass-coverage plan, rather than considering the needs and safety of the individual child. Timing of vaccines may represent another instance where your family's needs do not coincide with those of the vaccine industry. You do have a choice about the age at which your child receives shots, because the vaccine laws are linked to school admission, which may be at five or six years of age (except for those infants who attend day care programs). Delaying vaccination could be a significant step in your efforts to minimize the risk of adverse effects from vaccines given to your child.

A number of vaccines are commonly given simultaneously. This may create more of a burden on the system and cause a greater likelihood of adverse reactions than giving the vaccines individually. No studies have evaluated the effect on the immune system of single versus combined vaccines, but since vaccines have been shown to temporarily suppress various immune system functions, it is conceivable that combination vaccines could compound this effect (Jaber et al., 1988; Hirsch et al., 1981; Nicholson et al., 1992).

There is also some concern that combining vaccines could reduce the effectiveness of individual vaccines contained within the shot. For example, young children receiving the HIB vaccine may develop lower antibody response titers to the other childhood vaccinations when they are all given at once (Clemens *et al.*, 1992). If you feel that the administration of four to seven vaccines at one time could constitute a greater risk than giving less at each doctor visit, then this option might be one for you to consider. The problem with this option is that a doctor or clinic may not have the vaccines in isolated preparations, since giving combination vaccines spares the child more doctor visits and more shots, at the same time reducing the cost of medical care.

As the number of vaccines given to children continues to increase, the number in each shot continues to rise as well. Pharmacies have plans for the development of a "supervaccine" that will contain all of the recommended shots (ten or more) in one syringe. Their ultimate goal is to have this shot available at birth.

Table 3

Summary of Options for Your Child

Using some vaccines and not others

Delaying vaccines until after one year of age or later

Administering individual vaccines separately rather than
    giving them in combination

Individual Disease Incidence and Severity

The concept of parents choosing individual vaccines implies that they understand the issues surrounding the individual diseases. They must decide whether a specific disease poses a significant threat to their child. The factors that affect this decision process include the possibility of exposure to a disease, the severity of a disease if it occurs, and comparison of these risks to the possible risks of the specific vaccine. For some diseases this equation is simple, and for others it is much more complicated.

Chickenpox, for example, poses no health risks for a generally healthy child. The illness lasts longer and involves much more suffering in adults who may be susceptible when the effectiveness of the childhood vaccine wanes. It confers lifelong immunity, however, after children acquire the illness naturally. And the vaccine has potential adverse effects. Most parents will conclude that the risks from the chickenpox vaccine are greater than the risks from the disease. Other diseases, like *Haemophilus,* involve more complex considerations and sometimes more uncertainty.

Risking a serious vaccine reaction in order to prevent a mild childhood disease may not be the best alternative for your child. On the other hand, you may decide that preventing a potentially life-threatening disease may be worth the risk of the vaccine if your child has a significant chance of exposure.

Following the steps listed in Table 4 will enable parents to form an educated opinion about each of the diseases and their vaccines. Extensive information about the diseases in question and the individual vaccines comprises the entire second part of this book. Using these chapters, parents can evaluate each disease and the adverse effects of each vaccine. At the end of each chapter, a summary of the information also serves as a reference for quick review. Additionally, the information contained in the following general discussion of vaccine adverse effects can serve as background considerations to weigh in the balance when a choice is not perfectly clear about an individual vaccine. Your own philosophy about health care, your perception of the medical profession's reporting of vaccine reactions, your intuition, and a lot of information will establish a context to help you make these choices.

Table 4

Factors to Consider About Individual Diseases

1. Disease incidence and the likelihood of exposure

2. Severity and possible complications of the disease

3. Comparing the risks from the disease with the risks from the vaccine

---

Vaccine Reactions

All of the vaccines have significant adverse effects. These can be sep-arated into two groups: (a) immediate or short-term reactions that occur soon after giving a vaccine, and (b) delayed or long-term reac-tions. Immediate reactions include fevers, allergic responses, deaf-ness, convulsions, paralysis, central nervous system disease resulting in temporary or permanent disabilities, and death. Delayed reactions may be more insidious and less obvious. They can also result in per-sistent conditions that include epilepsy, mental retardation, learn-ing disabilities, and behavior disorders.

Adverse events resulting from vaccines may be due to the bac-terial toxin or virus component of the vaccine, or to the chemicals used in the preparation and preserving of the solution. These chem-icals include mercury, formaldehyde, aluminum, and a variety of other known toxic materials.

Vaccine reactions are notoriously under-reported. Many factors contribute to the reluctance of physicians to report a vaccine reac-tion, not the least of which is outright denial. Self-protection and self-reassurance are other psychological motives. Physicians do not want to admit that they have caused a problem. They like to think that their interventions are helpful, not harmful. They have also been assured and instructed by the vaccine industry that certain reac-tions that parents regularly observe, such as brain damage and death, cannot be attributed to the vaccines. A whole range of bizarre and pathological behaviors that infants display after they receive vac-cines must have another cause, they argue. It would have occurred anyway, regardless of the shot.

This type of denial and obtuse reasoning runs rampant in the medical literature. Case reports of severe vaccine reactions, whether published in the medical literature or reported to VAERS (the Vac-cine Adverse Event Reporting System), are ignored and dismissed. The generally casual, cynical, and paternalistic stance of the med-ical profession results in constant denial of claims for compensation for vaccine reactions, and absolute refusal to report adverse reactions.

Short-term reactions

Immediate or short-term reactions following vaccine administration have been consistently reported in the medical literature since vaccines have been in common use. Reports of these reactions have caused rebellion within the populations of various countries, and governments have responded in various ways.

In 1975, Japanese parents refused to give their children the pertussis vaccine after widespread publication of two deaths following vaccination. The Japanese government changed its policy in response to this protest, and delayed the recommended age for vaccination until two years. During the late nineteenth century, individuals in the United States protested that mandatory smallpox vaccination infringed upon their constitutional right of personal liberty. The issue was brought to trial and, in 1905, the Supreme Court upheld the rule that state police power included the need to protect its citizens from diseases. All cases since then have resulted in the same conclusion based on this precedent. When European countries began suspecting that the pertussis vaccine was dangerous, they eliminated it from the recommended schedule of childhood vaccinations. When parents in the United States have refused to administer this vaccine to their children, however, their children have been taken into protective custody by the state.

When vaccine companies began losing million-dollar lawsuits to parents with vaccine-damaged children, the United States government intervened and removed all vaccine manufacturer liability, assuming and limiting damage claims, and removing the possibility of any other compensation. This was the origin of the National Childhood Vaccine Injury Act of 1986 and the Vaccine Compensation Amendments of 1987. This legislation mandated that the Institute of Medicine conduct a scientific review of possible adverse consequences of vaccines. The Vaccine Safety Committee was established, and published two voluminous reports, *Adverse Effects of Pertussis and Rubella Vaccines* in 1991 and *Adverse Events Associated with Childhood Vaccine: Evidence Bearing on Causality* in 1994 (Institute of Medicine, 1991; 1994).

The Vaccine Safety Committee searched the literature, culling every report of a possible vaccine reaction. They found thousands of vaccine-reaction case reports and studies of adverse effects of vaccines in the medical literature. They reviewed the cases of vaccine-injury claims reported to the Vaccine Adverse Event Reporting System (VAERS), which receives approximately 1,000 reports of vaccine reactions per month. All of these reactions were catalogued by type of event and then evaluated by the committee. A judgment was made about each type of reaction associated with each vaccine, placing them within one of five categories. These five categories, listed in Table 5, refer to the likelihood that a vaccine can cause a particular reaction. Their conclusions about vaccine reactions dictate medical opinion, official positions, and compensation rewards. The weight of these judgments warrants some discussion of their methods and criteria for determining the relationship between adverse events and vaccines.

Table 5

Categories of Causal Relations for Adverse Vaccine Effects
Institute of Medicine, Vaccine Safety Committee

1. No evidence bearing on a causal relation.
2. The evidence is inadequate to accept or reject a causal relation.
3. The evidence favors rejection of a causal relation.
4. The evidence favors acceptance of a causal relation.
5. The evidence establishes a causal relation.

The Vaccine Safety Committee did an exhaustive job, citing every report available. They applied stringent criteria to these reports and studies, and determined that most conditions fit into category two—inadequate evidence to accept or reject a causal relation. The only conditions that earned a category-five rating, establishment of a causal relation, were:

- anaphylaxis (a sudden, potentially life-threatening systemic allergic response) caused by several vaccines
- polio and death caused by the polio vaccine
- thrombocytopenia (a decrease in the number of platelets, the cells involved in blood clotting) caused by the measles vaccine
- death caused by the measles vaccine
- acute arthritis caused by the rubella vaccine

The only conditions that earned a category-four rating, evidence favors a causal relation, were:

- acute encephalopathy after DTP
- shock and unusual shock-like states after DTP
- chronic arthritis after rubella vaccine
- Guillain-Barré syndrome after DT and polio vaccines

All of the other thousands of reports from countries around the world—from distraught parents whose children died within hours of a shot to physicians convinced that a vaccine resulted in meningitis, or deafness, or sudden onset of central nervous system disorders—proved inadequate to convince the committee that any causal relation exists between these events and the recently administered vaccines. Most types of adverse reactions reported in the medical literature and through the adverse event reporting systems were not recognized by the Vaccine Safety Committee as having a causal relationship to the vaccines. The list of conditions that fit category two, "inadequate evidence to accept or reject a causal relation," is embarrassingly long. That list includes 44 reported conditions and reactions that occurred following the 8 vaccines considered by the Institute of Medicine Committees. The list includes conditions with literally hundreds of reported cases—conditions such as meningitis and diabetes following mumps vaccine, and subacute sclerosing panencephalitis (SSPE) after measles vaccine. Other types of reactions, such as deaths from the pertussis vaccines, are denied. These conclusions are now used as guidelines in the award of compensations for vaccine-injured children.

Is there a problem with the Vaccine Safety Committee's findings? The charge of this committee was "the evaluation of the weight of scientific and medical evidence bearing on the question of whether a causal relation exists between certain vaccines and specific serious adverse events." The principle of proving causality occupied the majority of their deliberations. Simply put, they wanted to know if a specific vaccine *can* cause a specific adverse reaction, and whether it *did* cause adverse reactions in individual case reports.

This determination depended upon the concept of relative risk—the ratio of the rate of occurrence of the adverse event in vaccinated persons to the rate in otherwise comparable unvaccinated persons.

The question of whether a vaccine can cause a specific reaction could only be answered affirmatively if the relative risk ratio were greater than 1:1, that is, that a statistically significantly greater number of people suffered a specific disease or reaction soon after a vaccine compared to a comparable unvaccinated group. The greater the relative risk, the more likely the committee would attribute a causal relation to the vaccine. Therefore, the only way to establish a causal relation was to examine studies that observed the rate of occurrence compared to a control group.

They admit the problem: no such control group exists for most vaccines. "In controlled cohort studies, a defined group of individuals exposed to a given vaccine are followed longitudinally for the occurrence of one or more adverse events of interest, and the rate of such occurrence is compared with the rate in an otherwise similar group of nonexposed individuals. . . . In many populations, however, exposure to vaccines is virtually universal." They overcome this by establishing an arbitrary time period during which the reaction must occur: "Exposure can then be defined within a rather narrow time window; that is, the rate of occurrence of an adverse event within 2 weeks of vaccine administration can be compared with the rate of occurrence of an adverse event several weeks or months thereafter."

Who says that delayed reactions do not occur? The committee. Most clinical studies accept reactions within an even shorter time window than that. The vaccine injury table contained within Public Law 99–660, upon which compensation awards are based, allows only a 3-day window for development of encephalopathy (impairment of brain function) or residual seizure disorder following the DTP vaccine.

The strict rules governing the analysis of causation result in the rejection of most clinical case reports. If your child developed sudden seizures and extreme sleepiness within hours of receiving a measles vaccine and then experienced persistent problems with speech and walking, you would attribute the disease to the vaccine. You would have no doubt about it. The Vaccine Safety Committee, however, would view this report with skepticism because your child was not entered in a controlled study of adverse reactions. They have received dozens of such reports. Their conclusion reads, "Although there are a number of reports of encephalitis or encephalopathy following vaccination with measles vaccines of various strains, the rates quoted are impossible to distinguish from background rates. Good case-control or controlled cohort studies of these conditions in similar unvaccinated populations . . . are lacking. . . . The evidence is inadequate to accept or reject a causal relation between measles or mumps vaccine and encephalitis or encephalopathy" (Institute of Medicine, 1994).

When evaluating case reports of vaccine adverse events, the committee examined the following factors (and a few others) in assessing causality.

- *Previous general experience with the vaccine*—How often have vaccine recipients experienced similar events? How often does the event occur in the absence of vaccine exposure?
- *Alternative etiologic candidates*—Can a pre-existing or new illness explain the sudden appearance of the adverse event?
- *Timing of events*—Does the adverse event occur with the timing that would be expected if the vaccine were the cause?
- *Characteristics of the adverse event*—Are there any available laboratory tests that either support or undermine the hypothesis of vaccine causation?

In evaluating the available case reports, the committee adopted an analytical approach to calculate the probability of vaccine causation based on "likelihood ratios" for each element of the observed case. The likelihood ratio is calculated by comparing the vaccine as the probable cause to the probability of the same occurrence given non-vaccine causation. "The main elements of the case reports used in the committee's assessments included the individual's medical history, the timing of onset of the adverse event following vaccine administration, specific characteristics of the adverse event, and follow-up information concerning its evolution" (Institute of Medicine, 1994). Each case report was systematically reviewed, and very few could measure up to this strict protocol for determining causation.

The guidelines themselves predetermined that the committee would seldom find a causal relation between the vaccine and the disease, death, or disability that followed the receipt of a vaccine, no matter how many similar reports existed and no matter how quickly the reactions occurred. The reason for this is that an adverse effect would occur at the same rate after a vaccine as it does in the general population when the entire population has received the vaccines. This very complex analytical model falls apart because vaccinated children are being compared to the background population of vaccinated children. The frequency of vaccine reactions will be the same in these two equivalent groups, and the committee or any other vaccine researchers will call them "spontaneous events."

The other essential criterion for acceptance of a reaction involves the principle of biological plausibility. Simply put, this principle amounts to the idea that if science can't explain it, then we won't admit it. In the words of the Vaccine Safety Committee, "The vaccine-adverse event association should be plausible and coherent with current knowledge about the biology of the vaccine and the adverse event" (Institute of Medicine, 1994). If there is a biological model that makes sense, then that reinforces an association between the event and the vaccine. Lack of a biological explanation, however, may only show the limited knowledge we have of immune system mechanisms; not understanding it doesn't mean it isn't real.

Long-term reactions

Deep controversy surrounds the issue of delayed or long-term reactions, because these do not have a clear causal link to vaccines. In vaccine-industry jargon, they are not "temporally related"—that is the definition of a delayed reaction. For example, how do we know that the increased number of ear infections in a population of vaccinated children, or in any individual child, was caused by the vaccine? No one has studied this question. How do we know that the rise in attention disorders in school-age children has a relationship to vaccines? It would seem to be a logical conclusion, but no one has studied vaccinated versus unvaccinated children. Parents must make judgments in this area based on the experience of other parents and practitioners whose children and patients have not been vaccinated.

In general, such parents and practitioners agree that their children are healthy, and suffer fewer recurrent infections than their vaccinated counterparts. This may help reassure parents who choose not to vaccinate, but it obviously carries no scientific weight.

The other point for parents to consider involves the arguments themselves. The reasoned justification for the assumptions about delayed reactions may be convincing, and parents may have an intuitive response to these arguments. The risks from the diseases should be weighed against the risk of the vaccine reactions. These are reviewed in the sections on individual vaccines. In addition, there are theories that vaccinations are capable of initiating subtle and long-term damaging effects on the immune system and nervous system. These warrant some discussion here.

Critics of vaccinations have asserted that vaccines are capable of causing recurrent infections in children because they weaken the immune system. They say that the dramatic rise in ear infections, allergies, and asthma in children can be attributed (at least in part) to the damaging effects of vaccines. The incidence of asthma, the most serious and life-threatening of these conditions, has steadily increased in the modern era since the introduction of vaccines. Just during the period 1980 through 1989 the prevalence rate of self-reported asthma in the United States increased 38 percent, and the death rate for asthma increased 46 percent (Centers for Disease Control, 1992). Just in the five years from 1985 through 1990, projected estimates for asthma's medical costs increased 53 percent. The total estimated cost of asthma rose from $4.5 billion to $6.2 billion, or 1 percent of all US health-care costs (Weiss *et al.*, 1992). This dramatic increase has been attributed to increased exposure to environmental pollutants, and to the toxic effect of asthma medications themselves, but the increasing burden on the immune system caused by vaccines could also be responsible.

One of the most compelling arguments that points to vaccines as a cause of immune system dysfunction is the dramatic improvement that occurs in these cases following homeopathic treatment of the vaccine adverse effects. When a homeopathic doctor sees a child with recurrent infections, respiratory symptoms, or nervous system disorders which began after a vaccine, a common treatment protocol includes the prescription of a homeopathic preparation of the vaccine itself. This serves to antidote the adverse effect of the vaccine. Dramatic recoveries have been recorded in the homeopathic literature, including cases of immediate febrile reactions after vaccines and long-term illness patterns that resolved subsequent to the homeopathic treatment (Smits, 1995; Schaffer, 1995; Moskowitz, 1991; Moskowitz, 1983).

Several studies have examined the effect of vaccines on subsequent illness patterns in children to investigate whether vaccines can suppress immune system functions. The studies were stimulated in part by previous reports of an increased risk of acquiring serious invasive infections within the three weeks following receipt of the older capsular *Haemophilus influenzae* (Hib) vaccine (Black *et al.*, 1987) and the deaths of four children from invasive bacterial disease in Sweden after receiving acellular pertussis vaccines (Storsaeter *et al.*, 1988).

In two studies, no association could be found between the incidence of any infectious diseases and vaccines given in the prior 30 days (Davidson *et al.*, 1991; Black *et al.*, 1991a). These two studies evaluated children in the thirty days subsequent to vaccines compared to a control group of vaccinated children. Therefore, these studies are subject to the same type of confounding negative effect as other studies of adverse effects described in the previous section. One study partially overcame this deficiency by examining the incidence of acute illnesses in the 30 day period following vaccine compared to the incidence in the same children for the 30 day period prior to a vaccine. This study showed a significant and dramatic increase in nonbacterial fevers, diarrhea and cough in the month following DTP vaccine (Jaber *et al.*, 1988). Children had a higher incidence of illness after DTP compared to their health before the shot.

The ability of pertussis and DTP vaccines to stimulate the onset of paralytic polio provides further evidence that vaccines can promote serious disease processes and immune system dysfunction. Paralytic polio has occurred frequently following vaccination. This phenomenon was first reported in 1909. Scattered cases were reported over the next 40 years. Then, during the polio epidemics of the 1950s, series of cases of polio following pertussis-vaccine injections were reported around the world, in Australia (McCloskey, 1950; McCloskey, 1952), the United Kingdom (Hill & Knowelden, 1949; Medical Research Council, 1956), and the United States (Korn *et al.*, 1952; Greenberg *et al.*, 1952).

During a recent polio epidemic in Oman the problem of paralytic polio infection's onset soon after DTP vaccination occurred again. In this epidemic, 70 children 5 to 24 months old contracted paralytic polio during the period 1988–1989. When compared to a control group of children without polio, it was found that a significantly higher percentage of these children had received a DTP shot within 30 days of the onset of polio (43 percent of polio victims compared to 28 percent of controls) (Sutter *et al.*, 1992). The mechanism of this provoking effect of vaccination on polio onset has never been adequately explained, but it seems clear that an immune-suppressing effect of vaccines must be responsible.

Animal studies have also shown immune-suppressive effects of vaccines. For example, mice showed an increased susceptibility to infection following pertussis vaccine (Abernathy & Spink, 1956). Laboratory studies in humans have revealed evidence of immune system suppression as well. After measles vaccination certain lymphocyte functions essential in fighting pathogenic organisms are depressed (Hirsch *et al.*, 1981), and the number of lymphocytes, a type of white blood cell that fights disease, decreases (Nicholson *et al.*, 1992). Similarly, measles-mumps-rubella (MMR) vaccine has been reported to have a temporary suppressive effect on the function of neutrophils, another white blood cell (Toraldo *et al.*, 1992).

The *Haemophilus influenzae* (Hib) vaccine causes a decrease in measured antibody concentrations to Hib. This is true for both the older capsular vaccine and the new conjugate vaccine (Daum *et al.*, 1989). This depression of antibody levels is responsible for the early onset of Hib infection in the 7 days following Hib vaccine. Four case-control studies showed an increased risk of children developing Hib after receiving the capsular vaccine to prevent Hib (Black *et al.*, 1988; Harrison *et al.*, 1988; Shapiro *et al.*, 1988; Osterholm *et al.*, 1988).

The use of this vaccine was abandoned with the development of the new conjugated Hib vaccines. However, ten cases of Hib disease that occurred within 5 days after the Hib conjugate vaccine were reported through the Vaccine Adverse Event Reporting System (VAERS) between 1990 and 1992. Case-controlled studies have failed to show a significant increase in early-onset Hib disease after the conjugate vaccine compared to the prevaccine era incidence rate (Institute of Medicine, 1994). The Vaccine Safety Committee therefore rejected a causal relation between vaccination with Hib conjugate vaccines and early-onset Hib disease. Despite these individual studies, the weight of evidence in a large body of studies, cases, and laboratory findings indicates that vaccines can suppress immune system function.

Dr. Richard Moskowitz, noted homeopathic physician and outspoken critic of vaccines, has incisively proposed a possible mechanism for this effect. He suggests that the vaccine may be incorporated into the body's own cells, where it is capable of continually stimulating antibody production. Various kinds of naturally occurring viruses are stored within the cells of certain individuals and are associated with chronic diseases (herpes, tumors, panencephalitis). Vaccines could conceivably cause similar phenomena if they are stored within the cells. The constant sensitization of the immune system to the vaccine components within the body's own cells may weaken our natural ability to fight off other viruses and may cause an autoimmune response which could lead to serious problems.

> The latent virus survives as a clearly "foreign" element within the cell, which means that the immune system must continue to try to make antibodies against it, insofar as it can still respond to it at all. Because the virus is now permanently incorporated within the genetic material of the cell, these antibodies will now have to be directed against the cell itself.
>
> The persistence of live viruses or other foreign antigens within the cells of the host therefore cannot fail to provoke *autoimmune* phenomena, because destroying the infected cells is now the only possible way that this constant antigenic challenge can be removed from the body. Since routine vaccination introduces live viruses and other highly antigenic material into the blood of virtually every living person, it is difficult to escape the conclusion that a significant harvest of autoimmune diseases must automatically result (Moskowitz, 1983).

Our understanding of these processes is very limited, and the long-term effects of persistent circulating antigen in the body are unknown. It may cause a continual immune suppression, which disables the body's ability to react normally to disease. Certainly the continual reports of autoimmune phenomena that occur as reactions to vaccines provide us with incontrovertible evidence that tampering with the immune system through vaccination practices has led to immune system dysfunction, at least in the case of those individuals who suffered reactions.

The Institute of Medicine Vaccine Safety Committee identifies various autoimmune phenomena as well-documented adverse effects of vaccines. Many of these autoimmune responses to vaccines result in permanent, chronic disease conditions. The committee's report acknowledges the repeated incidence of specific autoimmune diseases triggered by vaccines that attack nerves and cause destruction of the nerve sheath (myelin). These demyelinating diseases, such as multiple sclerosis and Guillain-Barré syndrome (GBS), have plagued the vaccine industry. Reports of their occurrence following vaccination continue to pour in from around the world. In their attempt to explain the repeated occurrence of demyelinating autoimmune diseases that occur as reactions to vaccines, the committee members admit that,

> It is biologically plausible that injection of an inactivated virus, bacterium, or live attenuated virus might induce in the susceptible host an autoimmune response by deregulation of the immune response, by nonspecific activation of the T-cells directed against myelin proteins, or by autoimmunity triggered by sequence similarities of proteins in the vaccine to host proteins such as those of myelin (Institute of Medicine, 1994).

If autoimmune processes and immunosuppression caused by vaccines can destroy myelin (GBS) or joints (rheumatoid arthritis), then perhaps other destructive diseases also may have their origin in vaccination. This is the concern of various authors who identify cancer (Murphy, 1993) or AIDS (Curtis, 1992) as possible results of vaccination. Many critics have suggested taking a much more cautious approach to vaccine campaigns until we know more about these possible long-lasting devastating effects.

The possible long-term neurologic effects of the vaccines have been well-documented by Dr. Harris Coulter in his book *Vaccination, Social Violence, and Criminality: The Assault on the American Brain*. He delineates a hydra-headed syndrome of brain insult and injury possibly caused by vaccines. These effects include allergies, autism, dyslexia, learning disabilities, behavior disorders, and antisocial syndromes, all attributable to the assault of vaccines on the body. He postulates that vaccines have a damaging effect on the developing myelination process of the nervous system in children. This assault causes an allergic encephalitis (inflammation or infection of the brain) with widespread effects. That is, the allergic response initiated by a vaccine injected into the body is capable of causing encephalitis and brain damage, because the physical development of nerves is disrupted.

Coulter suggests that the developmental problems caused by vaccines occur in a large (and unknown) percentage of children. He speculates that the 50 percent of children who experience fever (accompanied by fussiness or screaming) after a DTP shot actually have a subtle form of encephalitis, and subsequent minimal brain damage. He points out the tragic irony of giving a dangerous vaccine to prevent disease-associated encephalitis, and achieving instead an insidious and permanent vaccine-associated encephalitis syndrome. His theories are based on the coincidence of the dramatic increase in the conditions he reports—autism, minimal brain damage, and learning disorders—since the introduction of vaccines. Coulter unequivocally blames childhood vaccines for the "new morbidity" of learning disabilities and behavioral disturbances.

> The physician is irresistibly impelled to characterize the "new morbidity" as "emotional" because these disabilities can then be blamed on the child or the parents. In fact, the responsibility should be placed squarely at the physician's own door. The vaccination program is intrinsically dangerous, which was never recognized or admitted.... (Coulter, 1990).

Coulter points out that no studies have been conducted to investigate the association of learning disorders and other modern brain dysfunctions with vaccines. The dramatic and immediate damaging effects of vaccines are denied by vaccine proponents. It is little wonder that wholehearted disinterest is generated by the possibility of long-term nervous system sequelae. Nonetheless, Coulter's arguments for a direct association between vaccines, encephalitis, allergies, and neurodevelopmental delays are compelling.

Chemicals in Vaccines

The chemicals contained in vaccines may be responsible for some vaccine reactions and adverse effects. Many toxic substances are contained within vaccine preparations, including chemicals used in manufacturing processes, toxins of the microorganisms themselves, and various impurities. The interactions of chemical additives contained in the vaccines with the toxins may also produce adverse effects when they are injected into the body. For example, the formalinization of crude toxins polymerizes impurities and other bacterial antigens, and these are not removed by subsequent purification steps (Relyveld, 1980).

Diphtheria and tetanus toxoids are prepared by extraction of toxin from the bacteria and incubation of toxin with formalin (formaldehyde) to produce the toxoid. This toxoid is then adsorbed onto an aluminum salt, and finally thimerosal (mercury) is added as a preservative to prevent bacterial contaminant overgrowth. Thus, the vaccine contains toxoid, formaldehyde, aluminum, and mercury—all with recognized toxicity—that are injected directly into the bloodstream. This section summarizes the potential toxic effects that relate to the chemicals injected with vaccine preparations.

Aluminum is added to vaccines as an adjuvant to promote antibody response. The tetanus and diphtheria toxoids, and the pertussis bacteria (DTP) are adsorbed onto aluminum salts (aluminum hydroxide, aluminum potassium sulfate, or aluminum phosphate).

Aluminum adjuvants themselves cause adverse reactions. Concern has arisen that the aluminum content of the DTP vaccine might play a role in the production of hypersensitivity reactions, autoimmune disease, encephalopathy, seizures, and neurologic damage by the vaccine.

One study showed the potentiating effect of aluminum on allergic reactions to pertussis vaccine. In that study, infants initially received either a series of aluminum-adsorbed acellular pertussis vaccine or a series of plain (non-adsorbed) whole-cell pertussis vaccine. When they were two years old, these children received a booster dose of aluminum-adsorbed acellular pertussis vaccine, and their responses were analyzed. The group that had previously received the aluminum-adsorbed vaccine had more severe systemic reactions (fever and fretfulness) and more severe local reactions (swelling and/or redness) in response to the aluminum containing booster dose compared to children who had previously had the plain vaccine (Blennow & Granström, 1989). The children in the first group (previous aluminum doses) showed production of IgE antibodies to the pertussis toxin, indicating an allergic response, after they received another booster dose containing aluminum. The group that had previously received the plain vaccine did not develop IgE antibodies after receiving a booster dose of either the aluminum-adsorbed vaccine or the plain vaccine (Hedenskog *et al.*, 1989). This suggests that the aluminum precipitated the adverse reactions and the production of IgE antibodies against pertussis toxin.

Other studies have shown that aluminum-adsorbed vaccines cause significantly more reactions than plain vaccines. In a Swedish trial of acellular pertussis vaccines, the systemic adverse reactions to aluminum-adsorbed vaccine were similar to those against placebo containing the aluminum adjuvant alone (Ad hoc group, 1988). Aluminum-containing tetanus and cholera vaccines produced a high incidence of local reactions such as redness, pain, swelling and abscesses at the injection site compared to plain vaccines (Saroso *et al.*, 1978; Collier *et al.*, 1979). This type of lesion in mice was caused by an interaction of aluminum and tetanus toxoid rather than by the aluminum alone (Goto & Akama, 1982). Some reactions to DTP may be due to this interaction between aluminum adjuvant and the bacterial-toxin vaccine components (Gupta & Relyveld, 1991). The toxicity of aluminum adjuvants has led researchers to seek other chemicals as replacements. Calcium phosphate is a normal constituent of the human body, and well-tolerated. Its use as an adjuvant has proved effective, as have the polymerized toxoids without adjuvants (Relyveld, 1980).

Researchers have discovered the ability of injected aluminum to persist in the tissues for weeks or years as subcutaneous nodules (Slater *et al.*, 1982). These tissue deposits from aluminum injections are likely to release the metal for many years (Crapper-McLachlan, 1991).

Aluminum has been implicated as a cause of **brain damage** and the accompanying symptoms of dementia, Alzheimer's disease, seizures, and comas. The association of aluminum with neurologic symptoms is especially significant, since the aluminum-adsorbed vaccines—diphtheria, tetanus and pertussis—have all been proven to cause these symptoms as well. The connection of aluminum to encephalopathy—the diverse range of neurologic symptoms caused by inflammation and destruction of brain tissues—has appeared in several contexts.

Aluminum deposition in the brain has been seen in patients with Alzheimer's disease (a form of dementia characterized by memory impairment, disorientation to time and place, and paranoid behavior). Aluminum has been detected in senile plaques in the brain (Candy *et al.*, 1986), in tangles of neurons in brains of patients with Alzheimer's disease (Perl & Brody, 1980), and in sections of different brain regions (cortical and caudate nucleus samples) of persons with Alzheimer's disease (Corrigan *et al.*, 1989). Patients with Alzheimer's disease have significantly higher aluminum levels in their blood compared to people free of the disease (Naylor *et al.*, 1989). Debate still surrounds the question whether aluminum causes Alzheimer's disease or whether aluminum accumulates in the brains of Alzheimer's patients during the progress of the disease (Eichhorn, 1978). A third proposed possible mechanism is that aluminum can under certain conditions trigger processes that are genetically determined (Eichhorn, 1979).

Exposure to environmental aluminum has been associated with an increased incidence of Alzheimer's disease and dementia. In geographic areas with a high concentration of aluminum in the drinking water, Alzheimer's disease occurs more frequently. This relationship surfaced in counties of the United Kingdom with high levels of aluminum in drinking water. Aluminum sulfate is used as a coagulant in water treatment, to help clear suspended matter. Most aluminum is removed during water clarification, but residual amounts remain. Researchers discovered a 50 percent increase in the risk of Alzheimer's disease in such counties (Martyn *et al.*, 1989). Similar findings have been noted connecting dementia with aluminum content of drinking water in Norway (Vogt, 1986). Another study showed that the relative risk for developing Alzheimer's disease was 4 times greater for areas with high aluminum content in drinking water (Michel *et al.*, 1990). A further study examined patients in an area of Newfoundland with a cluster of high rates of death from dementia, and discovered a high aluminum concentration in the drinking water (Frecker, 1991). Commentators on these studies have cautioned that other factors in addition to high aluminum consumption might contribute to Alzheimer's disease in these populations (Eichhorn, 1993).

The aluminum exposure from antiperspirants and antacids has also been associated with Alzheimer's disease. In a study that examined the relationship of lifetime exposure to aluminum in antiperspirants and antacids to the incidence of Alzheimer's disease, the risk ratio for Alzheimer's disease in patients who used antiperspirants was 1.6 to 3.2, depending on the frequency of use. For antacids the risk ratio was 3.1 to 11.7, depending on dose (Graves *et al.*, 1990). In another study, patients scheduled for brain surgery were prescribed aluminum containing antacids for 10 days prior to surgery, and their brain tissue specimens were measured for aluminum content. The patients who took a high-dose antacid had nearly twice the aluminum brain levels as controls (Dollinger *et al.*, 1986).

The neurotoxic properties of aluminum have been confirmed through several avenues of research. Tests done on primates have shown the ability of aluminum to stimulate convulsions. Aluminum applied directly to nerve tissue caused epileptic symptoms and persisted for years following the initial dose (Kopeloff *et al.*, 1942; Klatzo *et al.*, 1965). Aluminum injected directly into the brains of cats, dogs, or rabbits caused impaired memory and defective learning (Still, 1994). A single injected dose of aluminum causes first a disturbance of learning and memory, and then progressive deterioration of motor control, tremors, and seizures (Crapper-McLachlan *et al.*, 1991).

Aluminum is excreted by the kidneys when the rate of kidney blood filtration is normal (Recker *et al.*, 1977). People whose kidneys no longer function normally must undergo dialysis, in which their blood is filtered by a machine. When patients are exposed to aluminum in dialysis fluids, or when dialysis-dependent patients are treated with aluminum-containing medications to control serum-phosphorus levels, they develop a syndrome labeled dialysis dementia, or dialysis encephalopathy (Mahurkar *et al.*, 1973). Biopsies of brain tissue in fatal cases of dialysis dementia reveal high aluminum deposits in the brain (Alfrey *et al.*, 1976). The symptoms include incoordination of the muscles used in speaking, impaired short-term memory, tremors, spasms, and jerking of muscles, seizures, disorientation, and confusion (Alfrey *et al.*, 1972; Barrett *et al.*, 1975).

The findings regarding aluminum toxicity in dialysis and other types of dementia cases, and in Alzheimer's disease, point to the connection between aluminum and brain damage. The association between aluminum in drugs, in water supplies, and in antiperspirants with Alzheimer's disease suggests toxic exposure as a trigger for brain damage. The similarity between symptoms of dementia and seizure disorders noted in the aluminum toxicity studies and symptoms of reactions to aluminum-adsorbed vaccines suggests that it could be the aluminum in vaccines that triggers these adverse events. Aluminum adjuvants could play a significant role in these reactions. It is possible that the direct assault of aluminum, combined with neurotoxic bacterial products in vaccines, could not only be responsible for the immediate neurologic catastrophes of vaccine reactions but, over a lifetime of repeated injections, could also contribute to a cumulative deposition of aluminum in brain tissue that results in senile dementia and Alzheimer's disease.

Thimerosal (a mercury sodium salt) is used as a disinfectant. All toxoids, including tetanus and DTP, as well as hepatitis B and Hib vaccines, have thimerosal added to prevent bacterial overgrowth.

Many people have developed allergic sensitivities to thimerosal because of repeated exposure through vaccines. One study of unselected subjects found nearly 9 percent to be allergic to thimerosal on allergen patch testing (Schäfer *et al.*, 1995). A study of patients with eczema showed that 16 percent were allergic to thimerosal (Aberer, 1991). Other studies have shown that up to 37 percent of an allergic population undergoing desensitization treatment with thimerosal-containing allergy shots develop hypersensitivity to the thimerosal (Tosti, 1989). Individuals who are allergic to thimerosal can experience severe reactions to vaccines. Many cases have been reported in the medical literature involving apparent allergic reactions to the thimerosal contained in vaccines (Pierchalla *et al.*, 1987; Tosti *et al.*, 1986). It is probable that some unknown proportion of allergic vaccine reactions are due to thimerosal sensitivity.

- A 29-year-old man with hand eczema was patch tested for allergens. He was found to be strongly reactive to thimerosal. After receiving a hepatitis B vaccine he developed itching at the injection site, and 2 days later experienced an eruption of eczema that spread from his arm across his shoulder and back. This eruption persisted for a month and then slowly subsided over the next year.
- A 38-year-old woman developed a widespread itching eruption, beginning at the injection site of a hepatitis B vaccine. Eczema

and hives began spreading over her trunk, arms, and legs. Several weeks after the eruption subsided, patch testing revealed a strong reaction to thimerosal (Rietschel & Adams, 1990).

These sensitivities to thimerosal apparently develop as a result of previous vaccinations (Förström *et al.,* 1980). Even the minute amount of thimerosal used in vaccines (.1 to .01 percent) can specifically stimulate the immune system and cause sensitization (Aberer, 1991).

Mercury is a violent poison with many toxic effects. The toxicity of mercury varies depending on the form in which the element appears. Metallic mercury has different effects than inorganic or organic mercury compounds. However, major differences in toxicity are not expected among the different compounds within the inorganic group of mercury salts (Clement, 1992).

The group of inorganic mercury compounds includes thimerosal (an ethyl mercury sodium salt). These compounds are associated with a wide range of health problems, documented in humans and animal studies. The ingestion of inorganic mercury can be fatal to humans and experimental animals (Troen *et al.,* 1951). Lethal doses occur with large amounts of mercury salts (29–50 mg mercury/kg).

The kidney is one of the major target organs of mercury-induced toxicity, apparently involving the immune system. Several investigators have produced autoimmune kidney damage by administering mercuric salts to rats (Druet *et al.,* 1978; Hirszel *et al.,* 1985). Mercury has caused the production of anti-tissue antibodies with a specific anti-kidney activity (Hirsch *et al.,* 1986). Mercuric salts have also caused immune system suppression in mice (Dieter *et al.,* 1983). These effects may have significance for vaccine reactions, since many of the reported adverse effects of vaccines involve autoimmune mechanisms, and immune suppression is a significant concern in relation to vaccines.

The central and peripheral nervous systems are also major target organs for mercury-induced toxicity. Specific neurotoxic symptoms associated with mercury intoxication include tremors, dementia, and memory loss (Chaffin *et al.,* 1973; Davis *et al.,* 1974). These are the same type of neurologic symptoms observed in children following vaccination with the thimerosal-containing vaccines, DTP,

pertussis, hepatitis B, and *Haemophilus influenzae*. It is also interesting that the neurologic toxicity symptoms caused by mercury compounds have a delayed onset after exposure (Bakir *et al.*, 1973), which
may have significance for the suspected long-term neurologic symptoms of learning disabilities and behavior disorders associated with
pertussis vaccines.

Formaldehyde (formalin) is used to inactivate viruses and detox-
ify bacterial toxins. It is added to most vaccines and eventually injected into the body. Formaldehyde has carcinogenic potential in humans.
Exposure typically occurs through its use in the garment and fabric
industries, and contact with wall- and ceiling-insulation materials.

At least 28 studies have found evidence of cancer in people
exposed to formaldehyde. One study found an increased incidence
of lung, nose, and throat cancer in industrial workers exposed to
formaldehyde compared to a control group (Blair *et al.*, 1986). Another study found increased rates of nose and throat cancer in people
who had lived 10 or more years in a mobile home, especially those
mobile homes built in the 1950s to 1970s, when formaldehyde-resins
were frequently used in their manufacture (Vaughan *et al.*, 1986). In
several studies, risks of nose, sinus, lung, mouth and throat cancer
were found to increase in people exposed to formaldehyde (Ache-
son *et al.*, 1984; Olsen *et al.*, 1984; Liebling *et al.*, 1984; Blair *et al.*,
1990). The upper respiratory tract is particularly susceptible to the
toxic effects of inhaled formaldehyde. Nasal cancers have repeatedly been demonstrated in workers exposed to wood dust (Hayes *et al.*,
1986) and in rats experimentally exposed to formaldehyde (Albert
et al., 1982; Kerns *et al.*, 1983). Changes in the structure of nasal cells
have even been observed in beginning students of mortuary science
exposed to relatively low levels of formaldehyde. Those students were
found to have dramatic increases and abnormalities of nasal epithelial cells after performing an average of only 7 embalmings (Suruda
et al., 1993). Epithelial cell cancers represent the most common carcinogenic effect of formaldehyde (Swenberg *et al.*, 1980; Hayes *et al.*,
1986).

At least 19 studies have revealed an association between leukemia
and cancer of the brain and colon with formaldehyde exposure. A
significant risk for cancers of the brain and lymphatic tissues has
been found in most studies of formaldehyde-exposed professionals

(Nelson *et al.,* 1986). In a study of workers in permanent press garment facilities exposed for at least three months to formaldehyde, leukemia as well as cancer of the mouth were discovered. The incidence of deaths from these cancers increased with the duration of formaldehyde exposure, indicating a dose related association (Stayner *et al.,* 1988). A study of workers exposed to formaldehyde in a large chemical plant in Massachusetts revealed a significantly elevated incidence of death from colon cancer compared to comparable populations in that county (Liebling *et al.,* 1984).

Formaldehyde exposure following injection, ingestion, or inhalation has also caused liver toxicity and liver damage, as shown in several studies (Beall & Ulsamer, 1984; Stayner *et al.,* 1985).

Animal studies have confirmed the ability of formaldehyde to cause squamous-cell carcinomas (Swenberg *et al.,* 1980; Albert *et al.,* 1982; Kerns *et al.,* 1983). When bacteria, viruses, and mammalian cells have been exposed to formaldehyde, results included gene mutations, chromosomal aberrations, DNA-strand breaks, and inhibition of DNA repair.

Natural Medicine: Preventing and Treating Illness and Vaccine Reactions

The growing interest in natural medicine has been accompanied by a shift toward increased self-reliance, an awareness of the principles of self-healing, and the rejection of mechanistic approaches to medicine. Many people have chosen to pursue more life-affirming methods of health care that align with their personal beliefs about wellness, healing, and prevention. They view the methods of allopathic medicine, the pharmaceutical drugs, surgeries, and technological dependence, as things to be avoided. They find the concept of drugs used to prevent illness repugnant. If exercise and a healthy diet will prevent bone loss, why take hormones that can cause cancer? Why not rely upon natural methods to treat and prevent illness, when this is possible?

The return to low-tech approaches in health care has gone hand-in-hand with the concepts of recycling, using wind and solar-energy sources, and generally returning to a harmonious coexistence with nature. This is the philosophy that seeks to replace such obsolete notions as nuclear defense, clear-cut logging practices, and heedless toxic-waste pollution with more sensitive and sensible techniques. Similarly, the practices of water fluoridation, routine screening x-rays, and vaccination no longer seem appropriate.

The use of natural medicine implies an inclusive view of health and illness. The principles of homeopathy, Oriental medicine, and naturopathy place disease within a broad perspective. Symptoms and disease processes represent the body's signals that something has become unbalanced and needs to be set in order again. An infection indicates that the body's defenses need reinforcement. Recurrent headaches show that body systems need readjustment to return them to a healthy functioning mode. This may include adjustments of energetic body patterns through diet, acupuncture, physical-body adjustment, or the prescription of a remedy in the form of herbal or homeopathic medicine. The expected result is a stronger, more resilient body, less susceptible to the effects of stress or infections. Such an approach includes emotional as well as physical health.

In relation to infections, the natural healing systems of homeopathy, Traditional Chinese Medicine, and naturopathy all offer regimens for both preventing and treating diseases. Reliance on one or more of these systems should be the cornerstone of a natural approach to infection. These are the systems accessible to most Americans. Other, more exotic native-healing systems are probably just as effective, but generally inaccessible in our modern culture. Many other natural forms of therapy can assist the body in maintaining health. These include nutritional approaches, Western herbs, Ayurvedic practices, yoga, osteopathic manipulation, chiropractic, and a wide range of energetic and physical forms of massage.

Homeopathy and Traditional Chinese Medicine each have a long history of successful treatment of infectious disease. Long before the advent of antibiotics, both of these systems successfully managed epidemics and individual cases of complicated infections. The success of both homeopathy and Chinese medicine exists in sharp contrast to the helplessness of allopathic medicine when confronted with viral illnesses, and the ineffectiveness of antibiotics in commonly encountered childhood bacterial conditions such as whooping cough and ear infections.

Practitioners of homeopathic medicine assert that homeopathic treatment itself also affords some protection from disease. Homeopaths suggest that children who receive ongoing homeopathic medical care are less likely to contract serious diseases and will have fewer complications when childhood diseases do occur. Homeopathy claims to support the immune system's functioning, and the plentiful examples of cured cases of allergy and recurrent infection in children in the homeopathic literature support this contention. Since homeopathic medicines purportedly work by stimulating the body's defense mechanisms, proponents claim that serious diseases and complications of more common diseases are less likely to occur after homeopathic treatment.

Homeopathy is a system of natural medicine that has become highly developed and accepted in Europe and South America. In the United States, homeopathic medical care is less generally available, though it was quite prevalent and popular during the nineteenth century. Practitioners of homeopathic medicine have effectively treated the common childhood diseases for nearly two centuries. Homeopaths treated measles, mumps, and whooping cough during the 1800s, long before vaccines or antibiotics were available. Clinical studies have not been conducted to document the success of homeopathic treatment in these diseases or in the prevention of disease complications. Nonetheless, practitioners of homeopathy claim success, and express confidence in their treatments based on their 200 years of clinical experience.

Conventional medicine has little to offer when viral diseases occur, and non-homeopathic physicians are anxious to prevent what they cannot treat. The urge to vaccinate children is much stronger when adequate treatment is not readily available. Homeopathic medical providers, however, express confidence in their ability to treat viral diseases and prevent complications of most childhood illnesses. They tend to have less anxiety than conventional physicians about disease complications. If the diseases are less threatening under their care, then the impetus to vaccinate children is less compelling, especially when the potential for serious adverse effects exists in the vaccines. When parents in England who chose not to vaccinate their children were asked why they made that decision, more than

20 percent said they would rather place their confidence in homeo-pathic treatment of these diseases (Simpson *et al.,* 1995).

Historically, homeopathic treatment has proved effective in a wide range of acute illnesses. During the nineteenth century, home-opathy gained general acceptance because of its ability to cure infec-tious diseases. During the yellow-fever epidemic of the late nineteenth century in the United States, homeopathy was exceptionally effec-tive compared to the conventional treatment of the time. A report of the Homeopathic Yellow Fever Commission showed that in New Orleans homeopathic treatment resulted in a mortality of 5.6 per-cent of cases and 7.7 percent of cases in the rest of the South. This compared to an overall death rate of at least 16 percent (American Institute of Homeopathy, 1880). A comparison of mortality rates between homeopathic and conventional medical treatment in the United States and Europe in 1900 showed a two- to eightfold reduc-tion in deaths from life-threatening infectious diseases among the homeopathically treated cases (Bradford, 1900). During the severe influenza epidemic of 1918, homeopathic treatment also resulted in a significant reduction in mortality. These results led to a wide accep-tance of homeopathic treatment among the public. Although these studies were conducted in the nineteenth century, prior to the era of double-blind, controlled clinical trials, they serve as a landmark for the recognition of homeopathy as a medical science.

Clinical studies are once again showing the effectiveness of home-opathy—now in carefully controlled trials. Recent publications in major allopathic medical journals have shown the clinical effec-tiveness of homeopathy in hayfever (Taylor Reilly *et al.,* 1986), asth-ma (Reilly *et al.,* 1994), and acute childhood diarrhea (Jacobs *et al.,* 1994). A review of a large number of homeopathic studies published in the *British Medical Journal* concluded that, based on current research, homeopathy could be established as "a regular treatment for certain indications" (Kleijnen *et al.* 1991).

Homeopathy is a medical system that uses natural (plant, min-eral, and animal) substances that stimulate a healing reaction with-in the body and encourage a curative response to illness. This theoretical framework of cure is in distinction to that of allopathic or conventional medications, which suppress the body's reactions or kill bacteria. Conventional medicines are prescribed with little regard for their detrimental effects on the body. The benefit of the drug is considered worth the risk of side effects. Homeopathic practitioners claim that their medications have no side effects because they are so dilute. They are assumed to work because of their ability to trigger a reaction within the body; the medicine acts as a catalyst. The healing reaction manifests as a gentle and efficient cure. This has been the claim of homeopathy since its inception. Curative response, according to homeopaths, is not limited to the type of organism responsible for disease. It is assumed to work as well for viral as for bacterial infection. A single dose or a few doses of a homeopathic medicine are usually prescribed to trigger the desired response within the body. The minimal dose possible is employed to effect a cure.

Homeopathic medicine has several practical points which distinguish it from the methods of conventional medicine. A homeopathic medicine is chosen to treat a case of illness when it corresponds to the symptom pattern of the illness in the individual patient. Several different cases of ear infection or measles may require different homeopathic medicines. This is an important practical point: medicines are prescribed for the individual and not for the disease. The symptoms of the individual, in their details and qualities, are compared to the complex of symptoms characteristic of a medicine. When the right match is made and the correct medicine is taken, the curative response begins. In a serious illness, the medicine may need to be changed as symptoms change. The services of a skilled homeopath are required in order to make these decisions.

Homeopathic theory assumes that any drug treatment will either enhance or suppress immune system function. According to homeopaths, a drug will either have a strengthening or weakening effect on the body. Since homeopathic medicines are intended to stimulate the immune system, homeopaths claim that acute illnesses resolve quickly when the body's fight against the disease is strengthened by the correct medicine. The result is a stronger immune system, and resolution of the acute illness without resultant complications. In chronic conditions the body is purportedly encouraged by the appropriate homeopathic medicine to develop a higher level of resistance and less susceptibility to illness.

Homeopaths are generally concerned that antibiotics and vaccinations will suppress the body's fight against disease. Dr. Richard

Moskowitz has proposed that vaccinations may work through a continuous suppressive process. That is, the vaccine stored within the body's cells continually suppresses the ability to respond to a viral or bacterial attack (Moskowitz, 1983).

Several cautions about homeopathic medicines are usually offered by professional practitioners. Although homeopathic medicines are available without prescription, it is advisable to seek medical care from a qualified homeopath whenever a potentially serious acute illness occurs. Various combination homeopathic medicines are also available, labeled with indications for symptoms such as coughs, colds, teething, etc. These are not recommended, since the correct homeopathic medicine for the individual must be chosen carefully. It is unlikely that a medicine that is not appropriately prescribed for the individual case of illness will act curatively.

It is possible for parents to learn to prescribe for simple acute illnesses in their child. Several books are available to help guide parents in the proper use of homeopathic treatment at home. One such book, *Everybody's Guide to Homeopathic Medicines,* provides indications for the correct use of homeopathy in simple illnesses (Cummings & Ullman, 1991). It provides guidelines for safe treatment, and the appropriate times to seek professional medical care. Serious illness always requires consultation with a trained medical practitioner.

There are times when antibiotics or other medications are needed for infectious diseases, and a homeopathic or conventional medical provider can help make these treatment decisions. Tetanus is an example of a disease that requires vigorous, active treatment. It is mandatory that anyone who acquires tetanus receive conventional allopathic care and hospitalization. Similarly, any child who contracts one of the potentially serious diseases of childhood should be evaluated by a qualified medical care provider. He or she will observe your child for complications and the need for intervention.

Chinese medicine utilizes a complex theoretical system of understanding energetic influences on the body as its framework for treating acute diseases. The treatment of acute illness usually involves acupuncture and herbs. The purpose of this approach includes the encouragement of natural resistance, the dispelling of pathogenic influences within the body, and the harmonizing of bodily function. This system originated in China over 3,000 years ago.

The use of Traditional Chinese Medicine (TCM) continues in Chinese clinics and hospitals today in conjunction with allopathic techniques. In the United States, colleges of acupuncture and TCM have trained thousands of licensed practitioners to treat children's acute infectious diseases. Studies from around the world have proven the effectiveness of Chinese medical practice, and this record has led to the its recognition by the World Health Organization, and to the licensure of practitioners throughout the world. Parents who choose not to vaccinate their children may also choose to utilize Chinese medicine as a means of strengthening resistance to infection and treating acute illness to prevent serious complications.

A problem with TCM techniques involves the acceptability of acupuncture and strong tasting herbs to small children. Although acupuncture techniques have been developed specifically for children (Scott, 1986), and acupuncture has proven effective in treating children's illnesses, homeopathy remains a more palatable form of treatment for the pediatric population.

Naturopathic physicians (N.D.s) have been trained at four-year medical colleges, and have studied both homeopathy and Chinese medicine along with nutrition and Western herbology. They are well qualified to diagnose and treat childhood infections. An individual naturopathic physician often specializes in one area of treatment and utilizes other modalities as the need arises.

The Resources section (Appendix B) of this book contains information that will lead parents to find a qualified medical provider who can assist them in managing their children's illnesses and health care choices.

Treating Vaccine Reactions

The varied serious reactions to vaccines have no appropriate treatment within allopathic medicine, but homeopaths have treated these successfully for the past 100 years. Smallpox vaccine reactions were especially dangerous, and homeopathic medicine developed a reputation for its ability to successfully treat the sometimes lethal effects of the vaccine. A single homeopathic medicine, *Thuja occidentalis*, proved to be especially efficacious in relieving the symptoms that arose subsequent to adverse smallpox vaccine reactions (vaccinia).

During the nineteenth century the use of *Thuja* in the treatment of vaccinia as well as wide-ranging symptoms following the vaccine became a commonplace practice (Burnett, 1892).

Modern authors have found that the homeopathic preparations of the vaccine or the disease organism itself succeed more often in relieving the symptoms associated with vaccine reactions. Several case-review articles have been published which describe the successful homeopathic treatment of children whose symptoms began after the receipt of a routine childhood vaccine (Moskowitz, 1983; Moskowitz, 1991; Smits, 1995). Smits recommends using the potentized vaccine in four different strengths (potencies) over four successive days: 30th on day one, 200 on day two, 1M on day three, and 10M on day four (Smits, 1995). Unusually severe vaccine reactions may require a 30th potency, repeated hourly, for one to two days. Other authors have reported success with a single high potency (200, 1M, or 10M) of the vaccine. The dramatic recoveries reported following the administration of the potentized vaccine have led to a high level of confidence in the ability of homeopathy to treat vaccine reactions.

A preventive approach to vaccine reactions has been proposed by several authors as well. Smits, for example, recommends that the 200th potency of the vaccine be administered two days before the vaccination and repeated again after the actual vaccine. He further recommends giving the 30, 200, 1M, 10M series on four successive days, one month after a vaccine series has been completed (Smits, 1995). An American company under the medical direction of Rosemary Rau-Levine, MD (Celletech Ltd.) offers preventive kits composed of a combination of homeopathic medicines and the vaccine preparation in varying homeopathic potencies to be administered before and after the actual vaccine. These programs that purport to prevent vaccine reactions have never undergone any type of study to determine their effectiveness. Such a study would require large financial resources, and it is unlikely that any of these programs will be investigated. Parents who proceed with these programs should do so with the knowledge that these regimens are based on clinical experience and have not yet been documented according to the protocols of modern science.

Conventional Vaccine Studies

B efore considering each vaccine individually, some general points about vaccine effectiveness should be raised. Critics have charged that adequate studies of vaccine efficacy have not been conducted. The late Dr. Robert Mendelsohn, noted pediatrician, repeatedly questioned the use of any vaccine that has not been tested in a placebo-controlled or longitudinal study of vaccinated vs. unvaccinated groups. Very few studies of this kind have been conducted.

Public health authorities cite the decline in disease occurrence as proof that a vaccine works. In fact, most of the diseases in question have either steadily declined since the advent of general sanitation measures during the twentieth century, or gone through waxing and waning occurrence during epidemic cycles. Critics point out that a coincidental reduction in the number of cases following vaccine introduction in a community does not necessarily prove a relationship to the vaccine.

One set of statistics frequently used to document vaccine efficacy is the increase in pertussis (whooping cough) incidence when vaccine administration is stopped or decreased. This has occurred in Britain, Japan and Sweden (Cherry *et al.*, 1988). Many critics, however, charge that during times when the number of vaccine recipients decreases, physician sensitivity to the disease increases, and every lingering cough is then reported as pertussis, thereby inflating the actual number of cases (Coulter & Fisher, 1991). During whooping cough outbreaks, any cough that continues for more than 14 days can be labeled "pertussis" without a confirmatory culture (Centers for Disease Control, 1990). This is because the diagnosis of whooping cough itself presents problems and uncertainties. According to Moskowitz, the statistics of whooping cough incidence should be questioned, especially during supposed outbreaks when the population does not receive the vaccine.

> We should be skeptical about the "outbreaks" that are reported to have occurred. Pertussis, or "whooping cough," is actually rather difficult to diagnose conclusively, as it requires special cultures or antibody tests that many laboratories cannot perform and that many doctors, in the presence of suggestive symptoms, rarely take the trouble to order. Conversely, there are other cases of pertussis with typical signs and symptoms but no detectable antibodies. In other words, whooping cough as a clinical *syndrome* need not be associated with the organism *Bordetella pertussis,* against which the vaccine is prepared, or indeed with any microorganism whatsoever (Moskowitz, 1987).

This possibility of heightened awareness and bias also applies to the polio statistics during the 1950s epidemic. When the vaccine was introduced, dramatic reporting differences occurred, and cases previously reported as polio were now given another diagnosis, such as encephalitis, which appeared to make the vaccine seem more effective (see Polio chapter).

Underreporting of disease incidence also creates unreliable statistics. When the widespread use of a vaccine has lulled the medical profession into indifference about a particular disease, a large percentage of actual cases goes unreported. The Centers for Disease Control estimates that only 5–10 percent of pertussis cases are reported each year (Hinman & Koplan, 1984). These errors in reporting create unwarranted faith in a vaccine's effectiveness at preventing disease.

Vaccine proponents assure us that vaccines are safe because adverse effects are rare. This statement arises from the many studies which have investigated vaccine reactions. But the validity of these studies is severely hampered by two limitations. First, most of them have examined the occurrence of symptoms immediately following the vaccine's administration. Often this period has been limited to two days. Some studies have extended this period to a week or two. Any delayed reaction will not be observed in such a study. In fact, delayed reactions and long-term effects are difficult to document. For example, no studies have compared developmental or cognitive functions in vaccinated and unvaccinated children.

The second important limitation of these studies involves the control group. In all of the studies, the adverse effects in a group of children who receive a specific vaccine are compared to these symptoms in a control group, the supposedly "normal" population of children who will provide statistics on the "background" incidence of the adverse effect under consideration. The problem is that the control group is also vaccinated. If the adverse event under consideration is epilepsy or developmental delays, then the control group must be unvaccinated, because any of the vaccines may be capable of inducing these problems. One cannot compare vaccinated children with a population of other vaccinated children and hope to arrive at a valid determination of the risks associated with the vaccine.

Coulter has devised a list of criteria to evaluate studies that attempt to prove that vaccines are safe. In examining the incidence of adverse reactions, the authors of such studies can easily distort statistics through a variety of means. The task of evaluating an epidemiological study may be a daunting exercise in the analysis of research methods, but Coulter warns us against naively accepting the results of such studies.

> Because our medical literature is published in glossy journals, copiously illustrated, and with imposing rows of statistical tables, it may be difficult for the reader to realize that many of the articles are worthless. This is true preeminently of those about vaccination.
>
> For reasons profoundly rooted in the physician's psychology, and not unconnected with his source of income, the childhood vaccination program in the United States has taken on a sacerdotal aura, such that attacks on it are seen as blasphemous. And any statement in their defense, no matter how wildly inaccurate, is accepted at face value.
>
> Readers confronted with epidemiologic surveys purporting to show that childhood vaccines are safe and effective, should be intensely suspicious of the author's arguments (Coulter, 1995).

The list below provides examples of Coulter's criteria for examining the methodology of these studies. It is clear from these points that vaccine studies can be skewed through a variety of means.

- How was the sample put together? Is it truly representative of the population being studied, or were the children pre-screened so as to leave out those most likely to suffer vaccine damage? Were any dropped from the study while it was being conducted?
- If children are dropped from the study for having reacted violently, are they included as "vaccine-damaged" in the summary and statistics, or are they just ignored?
- How much "shoe-leather epidemiology" went into the study? Did the authors actually visit the children (rarely, perhaps never), or have they just shuffled Health Department or Blue Cross reports?
- Is the reporting system passive (you wait for the parents to complain) or active (you go out and perform a household survey)? The latter is viewed as a far more effective technique for disclosing vaccine reactions but, being more expensive, is less commonly used.
- How is a vaccine reaction defined? Is it highly restrictive (always) or generous and comprehensive (never)?

Coulter's conclusions are telling:

> My own experience with official American epidemiologic studies leads me to the conclusion that they are filled with half-truths, distortions, and outright lies, partly because of incompetence and partly because of the necessity to reach conclusions palatable to the funding agency. I once called this to the attention of a Public Health Service officer, and he replied, "That's true, but it doesn't make any difference; we already know these vaccines are entirely safe" (Coulter, 1995).

The problems with evaluating vaccine efficacy and safety are summarized in Table 6.

Table 6

Difficulties Tracking Vaccine Efficacy and Safety

1. Decline in disease occurrence prior to vaccine introduction.
2. Contradictory findings of vaccine efficacy studies.
3. Bias in reporting diseases when vaccines are begun or stopped in a community.
4. Deficiencies of studies evaluating vaccine adverse effects: observation period too short, inappropriate control groups, skewed statistics, etc.

Alternative Vaccine Methods

Conventional vaccines prepared by modern vaccine manufacturers represent only one form of disease-specific prevention. Vaccines and preventive medicines are also available to parents in homeopathic form.

There is a long history within homeopathic medicine of attempting to prevent specific diseases, especially during epidemics. This attempt originated with Samuel Hahnemann, the founder of homeopathic medicine. He used homeopathic dilutions of *Belladonna* to prevent scarlet fever during an especially virulent and deadly epidemic. In 1801 he published a short booklet about the management of scarlet fever, the first presentation of this preventive method to the medical world.

> Three children in a family had succumbed to a very bad attack of scarlet fever; the eldest daughter, who had up to that time been taking Belladonna internally for some other external disease of the finger joints, was the only one who to my surprise refused to sicken with the fever, in spite of the fact that she was always the first to catch any other disease that chanced to be prevalent. After that I did not hesitate to give this providential remedy in very small doses to the remaining children of this numerous family as a preventive ... and they all remained well and were not attacked in the slightest

> degree throughout the whole epidemic although among the
> most poisonous odors from their brothers and sisters, who
> were still suffering from the fever. . . . I concluded that a rem-
> edy which can speedily cure the beginning of an illness must
> be its best preventive (Hahnemann, 1801).

Since the time of Hahnemann, homeopaths throughout the world
have utilized specific remedies for the prevention of disease during
an epidemic. These efforts preceded the widespread use of vaccines
in the West. Edward Jenner, a contemporary of Hahnemann, had
just published his treatise on the smallpox vaccine in 1798. By 1806
the vaccination concept had spread throughout Europe, but enthusiasm subsided as difficulties with production and inoculation made
mass vaccine campaigns problematic and dangerous. Not until Louis
Pasteur developed more efficient methods of vaccine culture in the
late nineteenth century did the concept of vaccination become a significant public issue. Controversy surrounded the early use of vaccines and protests against vaccination thwarted efforts to conduct
large clinical trials.

In the meantime, homeopathic practitioners had success in preventing the spread of epidemics through the use of their medicines.
During the nineteenth century, the practice of using a homeopathic medicine that corresponded to the symptoms of a disease epidemic
became commonplace. The British homeopaths of the early twentieth century popularized this approach. Dorothy Shepherd and others published books for the lay person outlining the methods involved,
and many homeopaths contributed to the literature of epidemic prevention (Shepherd, 1967).

The medicines used in homeopathic form consist of two classes. One class includes those substances obtained from the natural
world of plants, minerals, and animal products. The second class,
called nosodes, includes substances derived from disease products,
tissue samples, mucus, pus from discharges, or pure cultures of
microorganisms. Nosodes correspond to the specific diseases associated with the individual bacteria or virus, or the infectious material
sample taken from a patient. Both of these classes have been used to
prevent disease. Examples of this include *Lathyrus sativa* (a plant) for
polio and *Pertussin* (a preparation of the bacteria *Bordetella pertussis*)
for whooping cough.

A medicine that has proven effective for a specific epidemic of a disease in the community can be used as the preventive for other cases of that disease, though homeopaths tend to use those medicines that have proven themselves in the past. As a general rule, homeopaths utilize the nosode of the infectious organism to prevent disease. Nosodes are named with the Latin terms for the infection or organism, *Morbillinum* for measles, *Diphtherinum* for diphtheria.

This method of homeopathic prophylaxis has been formulated into strategies and rules of two types—short-term prevention during epidemics and long-term prevention.

Epidemics

Experience with the use of nosodes during epidemics has led to a level of confidence and optimism about the protective effect of this method. Since the mid-nineteenth century, homeopaths have attempted to prevent or limit the spread of disease during epidemics, with some success. Most of the experience with this approach occurred during the era preceding the availability of vaccines. Homeopaths reported a decrease in the severity and frequency of disease in those patients who received the nosode preventively.

The evidence for effectiveness of this method is primarily anecdotal. A homeopath would experiment with a nosode during an epidemic, and then report that cases had been mild or infrequent. In this way, a level of confidence was established in the method. Clarke referred to the common use of *Morbillinum* and *Parotidinum* to prevent measles and mumps, in the Appendix to his three-volume *Materia Medica* (Clarke, 1925). He described giving the nosode in the 30th potency two to three times a day after exposure. Shepherd popularized the use of nosodes for epidemics that broke out in civilian populations during World War II in Britain.

The reduction or elimination of whooping cough vaccine administration in England and other European countries led to a greater interest in determining the effectiveness of the homeopathic nosode to prevent the disease. A study was conducted giving *Pertussin* 30c every three months during the first year of life, then an eighteen-month dose, and further doses on each birthday until the age of 6. Of the 1100 children in the initial project, 851 questionnaires were returned, and 694 of these qualified for inclusion in the study. Sixty-seven of these children (9.65 percent) contracted whooping cough during the course of the study. The rate of whooping cough among unvaccinated children in the same community was 27 percent during this same time period. This result suggested a greater than 60 percent reduction in whooping cough incidence in the children who received *Pertussin* compared to the general population. The author concluded that this pilot study provided justification for conducting a more elaborate study (English, 1987a).

The method of homeopathic prophylaxis has never been rigorously tested. Nonetheless, there is some evidence suggesting that homeopathic medicines do act to prevent diseases during epidemics. One study observed the occurrence of meningitis in a group of children who received a homeopathic preventive (*Meningococcinum* 10c in a single dose) during a 1974 epidemic in Brazil. Of the 18,640 children given the homeopathic nosode, 4 developed meningitis (0.02 percent), compared to 32 cases in the 6,340 unvaccinated children (0.5 percent). This represents a significant difference in a controlled study, although the control group was not randomized (Castro & Nogueira, 1975). Eisfelder reported an uncontrolled study of 50,000 children who received Lathyrus, a homeopathic preparation used to treat paralysis, in varying potencies during the polio epidemic of the 1950s. Only one of these children developed (non-paralytic) polio. The general population had a significantly higher rate of polio than 1 in 50,000 (Eisfelder, 1961).

These three studies do not prove the effectiveness of homeopathic prophylaxis in epidemics, but many homeopathic practitioners have been convinced by their own experience with this form of disease prevention. The practice of using homeopathic preparations to prevent disease during epidemic exposure may be effective. The medicines cause no adverse effects, and, in the absence of any other form of prevention, there was no reason not to use them. In an epidemic of a serious disease their use is still warranted, though there are valid reasons to allow children to undergo the milder childhood occurrence of measles, mumps and chickenpox to acquire lifelong immunity.

Long-term Prevention

Alternative vaccines in homeopathic form are available for long-term prevention. Several protocols exist for the administration of homeopathic nosodes or the corresponding remedies for the prevention of whooping cough, meningitis, diphtheria, tetanus, polio, and other diseases during childhood. There exists significant controversy within the homeopathic profession about the appropriateness of using these preparations for long-term prevention. This controversy involves the areas of effectiveness, safety, and ethics.

No long-term studies have been conducted to evaluate the efficacy of this form of prevention. There is no reason to assume that these vaccines continue to act preventively years after administration, unless immunity is shown through an objective test or clinical studies. The research that proponents of homeopathic prophylaxis frequently cite to prove an immunizing effect of these remedies involves studies done on diphtheria. An examination of this research is warranted because it represents the only studies used as evidence.

During the early part of the twentieth century, diphtheria research stimulated the investigation of a homeopathic preventive. Following the discovery of the first allopathic vaccine for diphtheria (Smith, 1909), a test was developed to detect immunity (Schick, 1913). The Schick test involves injection into the skin of a minute amount of diphtheria toxin. A positive result consists of redness and swelling around the site within 48 hours and indicates susceptibility to diphtheria. A negative test indicates immunity. It is also necessary to do a simultaneous control test to rule out false positive reactions that occur in response to other proteins in the test material.

The existence of this test for immunity provided homeopathic practitioners with a method to assess the effect of a homeopathic preparation used as a preventive and possibly as a safer substitute for the conventional vaccine. Chavanon published experiments in 1932 with 45 children using homeopathic preparations of the diphtheria toxin and observing its effect on the Schick test reaction. He discovered that *Diphtherotoxinum* 4M and 8M could reverse a positive Schick test result, supposedly conferring immunity (Chavanon, 1932).

In 1941 Paterson and Boyd conducted similar experiments using the Schick test at the Scottish Homœopathic Hospital for Children.

Of 33 susceptible children (Schick-positive) who received either the homeopathic diphtheria toxoid 30c (ATP, Alum Precipitated Toxoid) or the homeopathic nosode *Diphtherinum* 200, 20 children tested negative after the homeopathic preparations. This is a conversion rate of 60.6 percent of children from Schick-positive to -negative following the homeopathic treatment. Proper control tests were also performed on the opposite arm in this study, to rule out false positive reactions. No control group was included in this study, but when these results were compared to similar populations the shift in susceptibility from positive to negative far exceeded that of other groups tested. For example, a study of a similar population of schoolchildren found a conversion rate of 5 percent during the winter, and a conversion rate of 30 percent in a closed community of hospitalized children exposed to diphtheria (Dudley *et al.*, 1934).

These results led Paterson and Boyd to conclude that the homeopathic preparations caused a significant alteration in immunity, based on the conversion of the Schick-test response. They cautioned, however, "that nothing in this research is to be taken as indicating whether potencies of ATP or Diphtheric membrane may or may not have an action which increases the tissue resistance to Diphtheric infection.... Our experience of potency action on other lines would make us doubt that a long lasting immunity could be obtained by any limited doses of a homeopathic potency in the absence of the continual external stimulus of contact with a community morbidity factor" (Paterson & Boyd, 1941). These researchers did not conclude that the homeopathic preparations conferred immunity from diphtheria, yet several authors within the homeopathic profession have cited the studies of Chavanon and Paterson as proof that these preparations do provide immunity. They have continually used these studies as the only documented justification for homeopathic prophylaxis programs.

The question remains whether a conversion of the Schick test from positive to negative in itself indicates immunity or anything at all. The Schick test was used for many years as the primary determination of diphtheria immune status. It has been largely replaced by laboratory measures of circulating antitoxin in the blood because the Schick test proved to be a less accurate measure of immunity (Durbaca and Stoean, 1992).

More relevant is the fact that administration of the Schick test has been known to cause a rise in antitoxin titres (Ferencei *et al.*, 1969). Ferencei and coworkers tested the serum of 22 to 25-year-old subjects for diphtheria antitoxin levels before and after receiving the Schick test. They noted a poor correlation between Schick test results and antitoxin levels measured just prior to the test. More importantly, they found a significant rise in antitoxin levels following the Schick test. The accepted concentration level of diphtheria antitoxin titre that confers immunity is 0.1 IU/ml. (Bannister and Corbel, 1991). In Ferencei's study 21 subjects showed an initial titre less than 0.1 IU/ml. and 12 of them showed an increase of antitoxin levels to 0.1 IU/ml. or higher, five months after the Schick test. This means that the Schick test itself produced immunity that persisted at least five months after the test in 57 percent of subjects. Presumably a repeat Schick test given to these subjects would convert from positive to negative, if the Schick test reaction were accurate, which researchers in the field now recognize it is not. A total of 81 percent of Schick-test recipients in that study showed some increase in antitoxin titre 5 months after the Schick test. No cases of diphtheria were reported in this community during that period, and exposure to disease was eliminated as an explanation for the rise in titre.

Similar findings were noted in another study by Barr and coworkers, who measured antitoxin titres in the cord blood of babies born to tested and untested mothers. They found significantly higher antitoxin titres in the babies of mothers who had been Schick-tested (Barr *et al.*, 1949). All of these studies that question the accuracy and validity of the Schick test were conducted after the homeopathic research of Paterson and Boyd, whose study involved four repetitions of the Schick test. This repetition of the test could easily cause the results that they attributed to the homeopathic medicines. The recent studies would seen to invalidate Paterson's conclusion. If we throw out the Paterson study based on the more recent assessment of the Schick test, then there is no research to support the practice of homeopathic prophylaxis.

Homeopathic preparations have not been shown to raise antibody levels. Smits tested the titre of antibodies to diphtheria, polio and tetanus in ten children before and one month after giving homeopathic preparations of these three vaccines (DTPol 30K and 200K).

He found no rise in antibody levels (Smits, 1995). He speculates that protection afforded by a homeopathic remedy acts on a "deeper" level than that of antibodies. Other homeopaths have stated similar opinions. Golden says, "unlike conventional vaccines, the Homoeopathic alternative does not rely on antibody formation." He postulates that "Homoeopathic remedies reduce the patient's sensitivity to the dynamic stimulus of the virus or bacteria, thus lessening the patient's predisposition to being overcome by this stimulus" (Golden, 1994).

If homeopathic remedies do not produce an increase in antibody levels, then the only way to measure the effectiveness of homeopathic prophylaxis is through clinical results. This is a formidable undertaking. The cost of long-term studies using homeopathic prophylaxis would be prohibitive, given the present resources available. Ethical problems could also prevent such studies from occurring; it is doubtful that ethics committees would allow children to be deprived of the commonly administered and approved allopathic vaccines. Moskowitz has suggested that the sizable population of unvaccinated children whose parents have refused vaccines, could provide a control group to assess the long-term negative effects of vaccines (Moskowitz, 1985). Perhaps this population could also serve as a test group for homeopathic prophylaxis.

Golden has conducted an informal survey of customers who have purchased a kit of homeopathic medicines intended for use in a long-term prophylaxis program beginning in infancy (Golden, 1994). This kit includes the nosodes for whooping cough, diphtheria, measles, mumps and *Haemophilus*, as well as tetanus toxin and *Lathyrus sativa* (for polio). They are administered in repeated doses, one medicine at a time, during the period from one month of age to five years. For example, Pertussin is given at ages 1, 2, 13, and 32 months. Tetanus toxin is given five times at ages 11, 12, 24, 41, and 60 months. The first dose of each remedy is 200 strength, and subsequent doses are 200, 1M and 10M in succession, every 8 hours in one day. The follow-up survey involves a questionnaire sent yearly from 1988 through 1994, to each of the parents who purchased a kit.

During this five-year span, he received 879 returned questionnaires. Only 2 percent of those children contracted one or more of the diseases covered by the program. Parents were also asked whether a child contracted a disease covered by the program after a known exposure to one of these diseases; they reported that 188 children were exposed to one of these diseases, and 20 contracted the disease. This is an 11 percent failure rate for the homeopathic prophylaxis program with a known exposure to disease. Golden does not specify which diseases the exposure entailed. This very preliminary and limited survey suggests that the 188 supposed exposures may have received some level of protection from the program. Golden notes that symptoms were mild in the majority of cases that did contract the disease. No severe adverse effects were reported in this survey for any of the homeopathic medicines.

The only other evidence cited to support long-term prevention through homeopathy refers to the possible short-term protection it affords during epidemics. It is assumed that repeated doses may provide a protective effect that extends over a span of a few weeks, especially if the child is also challenged during this period with the microorganism that can cause similar symptoms to those produced by the medicine. There is no evidence, however, that any long-term effect accrues from this method.

Dosage schedules for homeopathic prophylaxis vary widely depending on the practitioner's preference. The schedule, the potencies used, and the number of repetitions are chosen arbitrarily. Golden devised his schedule to approximate the timing of allopathic vaccines, "to reassure parents that their children are being covered by a comprehensive program. . . . " Eizayaga employs 200c potencies of nosodes as homeopathic prophylaxis. His schedule involves giving one nosode twice per day for three days, waiting one week and then beginning the next nosode in his series. Others advise giving a CM (100,000 dilutions) once, or a 1M (1,000) that will last at least two years (Shepherd, 1967). In the absence of any studies or any way to prove immunity, homeopaths arbitrarily choose dosage schedules.

Disagreement exists among homeopathic practitioners about the safety of introducing a homeopathic medication into the body if there are no clear indications for its use. In general, homeopathic medicines are prescribed on the basis of existing symptoms. These symptoms guide the prescriber to the correct prescription. Classical homeopaths assert that an incorrectly prescribed homeopathic medicine can interfere with the action of other correct prescriptions or disturb the energetic balance of the organism. They generally do not condone the administration of many different nosodes in a single person, as some cases have been rendered apparently incurable by such practices.

Golden has addressed these concerns. He reasons that the damage caused by the administration of the homeopathic nosode is less than the damage caused by conventional vaccines. This is a theoretical assumption that may or may not be true. It is certainly true that homeopathic medicines have never caused the dramatic adverse effects including paralysis, epilepsy, and deaths that are attributed to conventional vaccines. Neither do homeopathic medicines circulate toxic materials in the bloodstream. He further states that the possible adverse consequences of protection using the nosodes are less than the probable adverse consequences of acquiring certain infectious diseases such as polio, diphtheria, and tetanus. Furthermore, even though he finds trust in the protective effect of a constitutional homeopathic medicine attractive in theory, this practice may not prove efficacious, since there are examples of strong and vital individuals and cultures who succumb to infectious disease. His conclusion is that homeopathic vaccines may prove effective, are less toxic than conventional vaccines or the diseases themselves, and are therefore preferable to relying on strictly classical homeopathic prescriptions (Golden, 1989).

Most classical homeopaths would counter that a strong and vital constitution does provide protection from the serious consequences of diseases, unless the disease is different than anything the immune system has ever encountered. Such may be the case with Polynesian islanders exposed to measles, or vital young adults exposed to HIV or the Ebola virus. Parents might also consider this possibility when evaluating needs for protection when children travel to foreign countries with endemic diseases that a child has not previously encountered.

On the other hand, most classical homeopaths will prescribe a preventive medicine or nosode during an epidemic, or following exposure if the effects of the disease could significantly compromise the health of the individual. This practice has some justification, based on the few studies that have been conducted, and on the considerable experience of homeopaths managing epidemics over the past hundred years. In most situations, classical homeopaths tend to rely upon constitutional homeopathic treatment and other immune-enhancing factors in a child's life to develop a strong immune system and prevent serious diseases and their complications, rather than experimenting on patients with unproven preventive medicines that could cause problems. Homeopaths cannot apply a double standard, assuming without any evidence that homeopathic prophylaxis can be used safely and effectively while at the same time criticizing the vaccine industry for exaggerating claims of conventional vaccine effectiveness and minimizing the recognition of adverse effects.

A separate question concerns the advisability of preventing childhood diseases if this will create a greater susceptibility and incidence of the disease in adulthood. Homeopathic prophylaxis results in the same situation as conventional vaccines in this regard. If the homeopathic program is effective, then these nosodes may require repetition throughout the lifespan to protect adults because they have not gained immunity by contracting these infectious diseases during childhood. Since the homeopathic medicines do not apparently act by stimulating measurable antibody responses, there would be no way to determine susceptibility to disease, or the need for repetition of doses. Therefore, the program might require repeated use of these substances on an arbitrary schedule to maintain immunity. Such a maintenance program would be as hopelessly speculative as the dosage schedule is now, since there is no way to document immunity.

The final difficulty with reliance upon long-term homeopathic prophylaxis involves ethical issues. Parents need to understand that there is no evidence to support the use of these homeopathic preparations for long-term prevention. A homeopath who prescribes a prophylactic medicine and assures parents that it will prevent a disease years in the future misrepresents the facts. False reassurance and wishful thinking may dispel parental anxieties about diseases, but they do not represent logical conclusions. There is nothing in the literature that even suggests that homeopathic prophylaxis provides lasting immunity from specific diseases. To claim that they do is an unfounded fabrication.

Some authors have suggested that if parents are given the choice of doing nothing or obtaining the conventional vaccines, then many parents will choose vaccines because they want to do something. Golden forcefully states his argument in this regard. He would "strongly argue that if parents prefer to vaccinate their children rather than provide no specific protection, we as practitioners are professionally obliged to offer them the use of the Homoeopathic alternative. It is then up to the parents concerned to choose between the two options for protection, based on the information available to them" (Golden, 1994). Homeopaths may or may not feel obligated to offer parents a program that has no basis in experience or research. If they do, the information should be accurate and not composed of contrived claims for homeopathic prophylaxis. The decision to use any vaccine rests with the parents. Nonetheless, practitioners cannot advise the use of homeopathic preventives just because they fear that parents will choose conventional vaccines if they offer nothing. This encourages the worst kind of anxieties, and defeats the purpose of a truly informed choice. Fear of disease has bedeviled allopathic medicine for centuries and has led to increasingly toxic methods of suppressing symptoms. Homeopaths would do well to present the facts to parents, and assume that parents have the intelligence and good judgment to come to their own educated opinions. Parents deserve to have access to all the information available, so that their choice about vaccines, conventional or homeopathic, can be an informed one.

Factors That Affect the Immune System

No discussion of vaccination would be complete without considering the factors that strengthen immune system functions. Several of these influences are under a parent's direct control. For example, breastfeeding protects babies from many infections.

The immunoprotective value of breastmilk is unquestionable, but incompletely understood. Immunoglobulins in human milk provide passive protection from bacteria. Specifically, secretory IgA found in breast milk blocks the attachment of *Streptococci* and *Haemophilus* bacteria to mucus membranes (Hanson *et al.*, 1985). White blood cells in human milk will actively ingest bacteria that invade the infant's body. In addition, lymphocytes carrying specific antibodies pass through breastmilk to the baby. Several other chemicals in breastmilk (lactoferrin and lysozyme) protect the breastfeeding child from infection by destroying or inhibiting growth of bacteria (Goldman *et al.*, 1982).

Many other resistance factors in breastmilk (including interferon) assist the child's developing immune system function (Chandra, 1978). It has been hypothesized that the high levels of prostaglandins found in breastmilk may protect infants from infections since prostoglandin E1 decreases inflammatory responses (Backon, 1984). Because of these combined factors, breastfeeding remains one of the best methods of preventing illnesses and their complications in infants.

Several studies have shown that breastfeeding decreases the incidence of acute illness in children. It is well known that in developing countries, infants who are exclusively breastfed have a decreased incidence of diarrheal illness compared to infants who receive supplements of formula, juice or water (Popkin *et al.*, 1990). However, even in modern nations with excellent sanitation, breastfeeding provides significant protection against acute illnesses in babies. One study of 237 healthy infants followed for three years found a decreased incidence of ear infections in infants who were breastfed for at least six months (Saarinen, 1982). Another study of 1,013 infants followed for the first year of life found a protective effect for single ear infections and recurrent ear infections in those infants breastfed for at least four months (Duncan *et al.*, 1993). A Scottish study of 674 infants similarly found that babies breastfed for at least three months had significantly fewer respiratory and gastrointestinal illnesses over the next year (Howie *et al.*, 1990). Most studies also show that exclusive breastfeeding is more protective than supplemented breastfeeding, and that the protective effect of breastfeeding for the first three to six months persists after children are weaned (Duncan *et al.*, 1993).

A person's nutritional status is another prime determinant of his or her general resistance. Malnutrition and undernutrition in underdeveloped countries contribute to low resistance and a higher prevalence of infectious diseases. Similarly, the introduction of refined and processed foods will lower the resistance of a population in a developing country and encourage epidemics.

Good nutrition lays the groundwork for a strong immune system in your child. This includes reliance upon natural foods, and avoidance of chemicals and refined products. Fresh fruits and vegetables provide essential nutrients for the growing child. Processed foods such as canned vegetables and jars of baby food have fewer vitamins, and altered forms of essential nutrients.

Babies should be fed cooked fresh vegetables rather than prepared baby foods whenever possible. The gradual introduction of solids in the form of fresh vegetables, fruits, and grains to supplement breastfeeding (or formula if necessary) during the second six months of life will help develop immune system strength and avoid the weakening effects of food allergies. Each new food should be introduced alone, to observe possible allergic reactions for several days before starting another.

The introduction of potentially allergenic foods too early in an infant's development may predispose him or her to allergic reactions. Avoidance of dairy products, wheat, and egg whites is advisable until a baby has been eating solid foods for at least several months. If a family history of allergies is present, then these foods should be avoided for the first year. Food allergies may predispose children to lowered resistance and frequent infections. The occurrence of chronic congestion or night cough, eczema, frequent colds or ear infections, or behavior problems are possible signs of food allergies. They should be investigated to see if this is the case. Avoidance of the offending foods, a rotation diet, or possibly homeopathic treatment will help the body to cope with the physical stresses of viruses and bacteria more efficiently.

Preschoolers and older children may not be the best eaters in the world, but if parents limit refined foods, sweets, and junk-foods, then the result should be a healthy body with a high resistance to infection. Children of all ages develop a sense of values about food. If parents set an example of healthful living and eating, then their children will be more likely to choose healthful foods. This is an important step in the establishment of immune system integrity and a lifelong pattern of wellness.

Most children love sweets, and these should be limited in all situations. Some children are more sensitive to sugar than others. They may develop symptoms of overactivity, distractibility, and poor self-control after eating sugar. Children often crave foods that stimulate allergic reactions in their bodies, and parents should be alert to these cravings as well as food reactions.

Parents should not underestimate their own influence on immune system functioning. The actions that you take can have a direct effect on the immune system. Diet, drugs, medications, and vaccinations all have significant effects. A good diet, avoidance of conventional medications, and the use of natural medicines that stimulate healthy immune system function will provide a good base for high resistance to infection and prevention of complications of illnesses.

Improved sanitation and living conditions have resulted in a steady decline in the incidence of infectious diseases and their complications during the past century. These changes preceded the development of vaccines. Long before the era of antibiotics and specific treatment of infectious diseases, the incidence of complications and deaths from pertussis, measles, smallpox, and scarlet fever had continuously decreased as a direct result of improved hygiene and sanitation practices. These factors are now taken for granted in the United States.

Overcrowding and lower standards of living in a community often accompany a higher incidence of infectious diseases and their complications than in the general population. For example, during the 27,000-case measles epidemic of 1990, over 45 percent of cases occurred in California. Over ten percent of these cases occurred in the San Joaquin Valley east of San Francisco, a low-income, rural farming area. One-third of these cases were in Southeast Asian children, 80 percent of whom were Hmong. It was found that a disproportionate number of these 352 children suffered significant complications (31 percent of these children were hospitalized and suffered a case-fatality ratio of one in every 29 reported cases). A case-control study investigating the reason for this high complication rate revealed that children from families with a lower standard of living had a significantly greater chance of suffering from severe complications or dying during this measles outbreak (California Department of Health Services, 1990).

Similar outbreaks of measles in inner-city populations of New York and Los Angeles accounted for over 30 percent of the epidemic (Centers for Disease Control, 1991). It is clear that lower-income populations with a lower standard of living remain at greatest risk during epidemics of childhood diseases. This was also proven in a polio outbreak that occurred in Taiwan in 1982. Even though 80 percent of infants were vaccinated against polio, studies of that epidemic of 1,031 cases showed that children were 5 times more likely to contract paralytic polio if they received water from non-municipal rather than municipal sources (Kim-Farley *et al.*, 1984). This epidemic provides further specific evidence that the level of sanitation rather than the vaccination level in a community fosters the spread of infection and susceptibility to complications.

Finally, mental and emotional health are a key determinant in resistance to infection. Emotional stress is associated with immune system dysfunction, lowered resistance, and more severe forms of infection. The immune system is enhanced in its healthy functions by relaxation, regular rest and sleep, enjoyable activities, and reduction of stress. These factors may be significant for today's children, who have busier schedules and increasing stress from academic demands and parental expectations.

We are now in a position to create environments for children that will foster emotional health and decrease stress. If we promote emotional resilience in children by increasing self-confidence and fulfillment, then a stronger immune system will be the reward. This can be accomplished in many ways. Children thrive when they receive positive reinforcement and praise for their accomplishments and growth. Children want to succeed. Love, attention, and encouragement are the parental tools that stimulate a child's well-being. Learning settings that foster exploration, discovery, and creativity will produce inquisitive minds. Strength of spirit and emotional well-being are associated with healthy physical development. Children who feel confident, strong, and happy are more likely to have an efficient immune system.

Legal
Requirements

In civilized countries vaccines are optional and free.

It continually amazes me that more parents do not avail themselves of exemptions from vaccines. Most parents that I interview mistakenly believe that without vaccines their children will not be admitted to school. The school districts, the medical profession, and the media perpetuate this myth. Parents who question the use of vaccines usually receive harsh accusations and bullying tactics from their pediatrician, and relent under this intimidating onslaught. They decide that the issue is not worth the fight and the alienation of their child's doctor. It is usually not laws that force parents to vaccinate, but the professionals, both medical and educational, who care for their child.

The United States government also takes the vaccine campaign very seriously. Parents who make an informed choice about vaccines for their children must contend with compulsory vaccine laws. Conscientious objection to these laws is not handled liberally by the courts. In 1905 the Supreme Court ruled that an individual could not refuse the smallpox vaccine on constitutional grounds of infringement on personal liberty. The court found that an individual's personal liberty must give way to the state's protection of other citizens' health (*Jacobson v. Massachusetts,* 197 US 11, 25; 1905).

Since that time, various state courts have ruled that compulsory immunization statutes cannot be stricken down on constitutional grounds. Every state has a compulsory vaccination law, though the specific requirements for individual vaccines vary from state to state. This means that parents or legal guardians who decide not to give the vaccines will need to seek a legal exemption from vaccines. These come in three varieties: medical, religious, and philosophical. Not all states have philosophical exemptions, so parents in those states must seek either a religious or medical exemption. Usually the issue of a child's unvaccinated status will arise upon registration for school or day care. Schools require an immunization record, and parents must have proof that their child has been vaccinated, signed by a health care provider. Schools become involved in the vaccination campaign because state and local governments receive federal funding for immunization programs. The federal Public Health Service Act, 42 U.S.C. § 262 requires that participating governments must have a "... plan to assure that children begin and complete their immunizations on schedule ..." and "a plan to systematically immunize susceptible children at school entry through vigorous enforcement of school immunization laws" (42 C.F.R. § 5lb.204).

Other situations that may draw attention to an unvaccinated child are visits to an emergency room, clinic, or doctor's office. Parents inform the doctor that the child has not been vaccinated, or they refuse vaccination, and the doctor files a report. When confronted with one of these situations, the parents then seek an exemption. When the exemption is accepted by the school or the health department, the issue is resolved. If a request for exemption is denied, then parents may appeal that decision.

Parents who continue to have difficulty with school and governmental authorities may need to seek legal counsel. One attorney has advised the following legal tactic to avoid litigation if a school continues to refuse admission or if authorities question the parents' legal right to refuse vaccines:

> Some attorneys have successfully prevented litigation by demanding from the school board, the hospital, and the physician administering the vaccine a guarantee that the vaccine will not cause disease, death or injurious side effects. The guarantee usually states that the vaccine will prevent the particular disease for which it is given. It is worded in such a way so as to make the persons signing it not only liable as a

representative of the school district or hospital but also individually for damages should any damage in fact occur. To my knowledge no one has ever signed such a document and in each case in which it was used the child has been allowed to return to class without the vaccination (Finn, 1983).

Medical Exemptions

All fifty states provide for medical exemption from vaccines. If a physician thinks a child should not have the vaccine, then he or she can provide an exemption. Many doctors are willing to write these, especially if they think the vaccines may have unknown long-term effects that could be detrimental to your child's health. The pediatric literature lists specific medical contraindications for the various vaccines. These conditions are either quite limited in scope (e.g., recent onset of a neurologic disorder or prior serious reaction to the vaccine), or include temporary situations such as an acute illness or a fever.

Physicians may consider themselves at risk if they provide an exemption for any other reason than those on the official lists. One such case was reported by the Centers for Disease Control. A 12-year-old boy acquired tetanus from a splinter and recovered after twelve days of hospitalization. The report was titled, "Tetanus in a Child with Improper Medical Exemption from Immunization—Florida."

> Investigation revealed that the child had received a dose of oral polio vaccine at about 18 months of age but had received no other immunizations. In the school record was a form granting him permanent medical exemption to all vaccines. The form, signed by a health-care provider, gave the reason for exemption as "due to recent medical literature." The provider later stated that the literature referred to "cytotoxic allergies secondary to immunization," but cited no specific references. Review of immunization records in the child's school revealed two other children with similar exemptions granted by this same provider.

They caution that "granting of medical exemptions should not be given indiscriminately." A poor choice of English, but such a notice serves as an undisguised warning to the medical profession (Centers for Disease Control, 1985). Medical exemptions have been more carefully scrutinized since the most recent vaccine campaigns of the 1990s.

Wording of the medical exemption is not standardized. A physician can state anything appropriate to the individual child. A simple statement that vaccines are waived indefinitely because of potential adverse effects may suffice. The following alternate wording may help to limit the liability of a health care provider and still release the parents from immunization requirements.

> In the opinion of the parents, vaccines would be inadvisable at this time from a medical perspective. Informed consent was not given for this procedure because of a history of allergic reactions (or low tolerance to medications).

Additionally, the following statement may be added as a verification of the parents' commitment to their decision.

> It is the parents' sincere conviction that vaccine administration would be an invasion of the body's integrity.

Parents who think that their child's medical condition warrants exemption from vaccines should consult an attorney who specializes in this area. Obtaining a medical exemption for a child with a chronic illness may involve complex considerations. An attorney can advise parents concerning case precedent and the best tactics for making the legal argument necessary to obtain a valid medical exemption.

Religious Exemptions

All states except Mississippi and West Virginia allow exemption from vaccination on the basis of parents' religious beliefs. Parents may be members of a religious organization that opposes the use of vaccines, or they can claim an exemption based on their personal religious beliefs that are similar to those of such an organization. Recent legal precedents have established that exemptions should be granted on the basis of parents' personal religious beliefs, and that parents need not be associated with a religious institution opposed to vaccination. These cases have established that the religious exemption must extend to individuals who hold sincere religious convictions against the use of vaccines, and that these convictions may be broad in scope. Religious belief, in other words, need not conform to a specific religion but can encompass spiritual convictions such as a pantheistic view of creative energy in the universe, or beliefs that bear a similarity to those of Eastern religions or Native American traditions.

Several court cases have established that personal religious belief qualifies parents for a religious exemption. School districts and state education departments have lost monetary damage suits for depriving children of their rights to public education when they were denied a religious exemption (*Sherr and Levy v. Northport-East Northport Union Free School District*, 672 F. Supp. 81; E.D.N.Y. 1987). The Massachusetts Supreme Court held that the law granting exemptions to members of a religion that opposed vaccines must also apply to individuals with the same religious beliefs, regardless of their affiliation with a church. The court decided that the law could not grant such preference to certain religious groups (*Dalli v. Board of Education*, 358 Mass. 753, 1971). A similar case in New York found that personal religious beliefs held by the parents constituted grounds for granting an exemption even though the parents did not belong to a church or hold beliefs advocated by any specific religion (*Allanson v. Clinton School District*, No. CV 84–174, slip op. at 5, N.D.N.Y. 1984).

Parents seeking a religious exemption need to submit a letter to the school stating their desire for a waiver of vaccines based on their religious belief. The wording of such a letter is important, and should conform to the wording of the statute governing exemptions. It should also state the parents' sincere beliefs, related in such a way that they can be interpreted by the court as religious. The wording of the immunization law can be obtained from the state health-department's immunization office.

Parents seeking such an exemption should contact an attorney who specializes in immunization law. They must construct a solid legal case based on their individual situation, their state law, and their own beliefs. Since religious belief can be interpreted broadly, a wide range of personal beliefs and philosophies will qualify parents for a religious exemption. The case that is constructed in the letter must conform to the legal arguments that will be used in litigation if the school and state government authorities reject the parents' petition for exemption. A well-constructed case and an attorney's arguments will usually prevent litigation. The small cost of involving an attorney early in this process will help prevent the major expense of going to court later.

The vaccine campaign and government pressure to vaccinate all children have made schools wary about granting religious exemptions. This is a legal issue of personal choice. If schools deny parents their legal rights, then an attorney will challenge that infringement in a court of law. This is the message that a legal argument will convey to the school district and the state government.

Parents confronted with a denial of their legal rights should not acquiesce because of harassment or intimidation. The law is on your side, and it is not in the school's financial interest to pursue litigation. Letters from an attorney can be very persuasive. All communications should be in writing. Document any phone conversations. Since the common goal of the parents and the school district is to educate the child and abide by the law, a solution to a dispute over vaccine exemption can usually be reached through logic and an appropriate review of the legal requirements. The school must abide by the law.

The medical establishment has repeatedly sought to eliminate the religious exemption on constitutional grounds and through legislation. For example, a federal court case was filed in 1993 on behalf of the California Medical Association (CMA) against the United States Government. The CMA argued that the court should not allow children to be deprived of medical care in the form of vaccinations because their parents withhold consent; that this would be in violation of a child's right to liberty secured by the Fourteenth Amendment to the Constitution, which guarantees that "No State shall make or enforce any law which shall abridge the privileges or immunities of citizens of the United States; nor shall any State deprive any person of life, liberty, or property, without due process of law." The CMA claimed that, "Parents must not be free to expose their children to deleterious health conditions.... A child's constitutional right to develop fully must be protected.... In fact, the Court has specified that the right to practice religion freely does not include the liberty to expose the community or a child to ill health or death."

They quoted a case precedent to bolster their argument (*Prince*, 321 US at 170). "Elaborating on the issue of parental autonomy, the

Court in *Prince* stated: 'Parents may be free to become martyrs themselves. But it does not follow they are free in identical circumstances, to make martyrs of their children before they have reached the age of full and legal discretion when they can make that choice for themselves.'" They requested that the court address "the question of the constitutionality of the religious exemptions provisions currently contained in California child welfare legislation and to hold those provisions constitutionally invalid" (California Medical Association, 1993). Presumably this argument is based on the principle of *"Parens Patriae."* As explained by an attorney who specializes in vaccine law, this doctrine provides for the ability of States to "compel medical treatment necessary to preserve the life or health of a minor citizen notwithstanding vehement parental objection. With its usual deference to the integrity of the family unit and the notion of parental control of minors, the State exercises its power narrowly" (Finn, 1983).

The CMA case was dismissed by the US Court of Appeals in 1994 because of the many case precedents upholding the right of religious exemption, but this challenge to exemptions is not an isolated event. The vaccine industry will continue its attempts to curtail parental rights to make informed health care choices for their children. Similarly, legislation is periodically proposed in various states to eliminate religious and philosophical exemptions from vaccines. These undisguised and unpublicized efforts to limit parents' choices and to undermine parents' fundamental rights continually reveal the motives of the vaccine industry as the guarantee of massive sales and enforced belief in vaccines.

Philosophical Exemptions

Nineteen states provide the option of personal or philosophical belief exemptions (See Table 7). This means that parents need not justify their preference for avoiding vaccines except to say that they are philosophically opposed to their children receiving them. Parents residing in states that provide a philosophical exemption must sign a form or write a letter that says immunization is contrary to their beliefs. Some states provide a waiver statement on the school district immunization record forms included with registration materials.

Other states require a written statement from the parents. Parents need only request the immunization exemption form at their school district office when enrolling their child in school, or present the school district a simple letter.

Table 7

States that Allow a Philosophical Exemption from Vaccination

Arizona	Nebraska
California	New Mexico
Colorado	North Dakota
Idaho	Ohio
Indiana	Oklahoma
Louisiana	Rhode Island
Maine	Utah
Michigan	Vermont
Minnesota	Washington
	Wisconsin

(US Dept. of Health and Human Services, *State Immunization Requirements* 1993–1994)

Private schools can set their own requirements for admission. Day care centers, preschools, nursery schools and private schools can refuse admission to a child for a variety of reasons. Most of these facilities, however, are willing to abide by the recommendations of state health departments concerning immunization requirements, and some states include these day care and private educational facilities within the statute. A physician's medical exemption should be an adequate waiver in all states, and in states with provisions for religious or philosophical exemptions a parent's signed statement should suffice.

If the director of a private school or day care center is hesitant about admitting your child, then he or she should be encouraged to contact the medical director of immunizations at the state health department. Refusal to admit a child on the basis of "inadequate" immunization could create a legal liability for a private school in a state where religious or philosophical exemptions exist. That is, parents could take a school to court if the school refuses admission to their child in a state with personal belief exemptions.

Table 8

States That Do Not Require Pertussis Vaccination for Grades K–12

Idaho	Oregon
Maine	Pennsylvania
Missouri	Texas
New York	Washington

Many attorneys and individuals are working to ensure freedom of choice in the area of child vaccination. One organization in particular, Dissatisfied Parents Together (DPT), has been instrumental in the passage of legislation that protects children and their parents (see Appendix B: Resources). If a parent makes the choice to avoid a required vaccine, then support for that decision is available.

Options for Legal Exemption from Vaccines

1. Use the philosophical belief exemption, if available in your state;
2. Find a doctor willing to write a medical exemption; or
3. Develop a personal legal case for religious exemption, with the help of an attorney.

PART II

The Vaccines

The Diseases
and Their Vaccines

The following chapters discuss individual diseases and the vaccines currently recommended for children in the United States by the Centers for Disease Control. I present a brief summary of each disease, its corresponding vaccine, and the critical factors surrounding its use. I have included information about disease incidence, vaccine efficacy, and adverse reactions to vaccines because these figures are not readily available to the general public. Statistics concerning disease incidence always refer to the United States unless specifically stated otherwise.

Each section includes many references to the medical literature because I feel parents should have facts about vaccines and not just opinions and official recommendations. Our knowledge about vaccines is limited, but parents need to be involved in the controversy that this partial picture generates. This technical information is summarized in tables at the end of each section. I have used original citations from the medical literature—doctors speaking to other doctors. This is not the picture that parents usually encounter at their pediatrician's office where a rosy light is shed upon vaccination.

All vaccines have problems with toxicity and adverse effects, ineffectiveness, and contamination. Full disclosure occurs nowhere—not in the pediatrician's office, not in the pharmaceutical inserts, and not in the medical literature. I have collected it here to allow parents an undisguised view of vaccines. Not all reported cases of adverse reactions to vaccines can actually be attributed to the vaccine. Some symptoms unrelated to vaccines will occur coincidentally following vaccination, and these may be reported in studies along with actual vaccine reactions. The weight of evidence will determine whether a certain effect is caused by the vaccine. I have included the majority of reports for each vaccine so that parents can see the weight of that evidence for themselves.

There is no question that the incidence of individual diseases has declined, at least in part, because of vaccination. But the cost in adverse effects from vaccines may be too high for us to tolerate given our present level of knowledge about the vaccines and disease occurrence. I have included my own recommendations for vaccine use, so parents will know my opinion and conclusions about the vaccines. Ultimately, the choice for your child rests with you.

Tetanus

The disease that parents usually worry about most is tetanus. Unlike the other diseases discussed in this book, tetanus is caused by a microorganism that enters the skin through a wound. Tetanus is potentially fatal, and it strikes otherwise healthy individuals. The repeated exposure of young children to cuts, scrapes, and dirt provides a continual source of anxiety for parents of unvaccinated children. The organism responsible for tetanus is found in soil and the intestinal tracts of farm animals. Any manure-treated soil may be infectious.

The symptoms of tetanus begin with stiffness of muscles; the muscles of the jaw and neck are the first to be involved. In the 24 to 48 hours after onset of the disease, muscle rigidity may be fully developed and involve the trunk and extremities. The neck and back become stiff and arched, and the abdomen board-like. Painful spasms can be produced by the slightest stimulant (noise, touch, light), and it is spasms of the respiratory muscles that cause asphyxia and death.

The incubation period for tetanus varies from one day to three weeks, although the usual range is one to two weeks. There is no sign of tetanus in the wound itself, and usually no symptoms until the muscle stiffness begins. Fever is generally low-grade or absent, and the senses remain clear.

Treatment for tetanus is drastic. Muscle relaxants, sedatives, antibiotics, immune globulin, and antitoxins are administered. The person is put in a low-stimulus environment and often fed through a stomach tube, and an artificial airway may be required during treatment. There is no effective alternative treatment.

Incidence

The following statistics will help to put the tetanus problem into perspective. Since 1976 there have been less than 100 cases of tetanus per year in the United States (Centers for Disease Control, 1994). The majority of these cases are people over age 50, and tetanus is now recognized as primarily a disease of older adults in the US. On average 5 percent or less of tetanus cases occur in individuals less than 20 years of age (Centers for Disease Control, 1987). The case-fatality ratio for individuals less than 50 years old is less than 5 percent. In other words, only a few cases of tetanus occur each year in children, and these are very rarely fatal.

During 1993 no cases of tetanus occurred in children. Of the 48 total tetanus cases reported in 1993, 34 (70 percent) occurred in individuals over 50 years old (Centers for Disease Control, 1994). The total case-fatality ratio is approximately 30 percent (Centers for Disease Control, 1987). The higher distribution of tetanus cases among the elderly is generally attributed to the low rate of tetanus vaccination among this group. Eighty-seven percent of children at two years old have received a primary series of tetanus vaccine injections (Centers for Disease Control, 1994a). By contrast, serosurveys indicate that one-half to two-thirds of persons 60 or older lack protective levels of circulating antitoxin antibody against tetanus (Centers for Disease Control, 1985). The high percentage of vaccinated children is at least partially responsible for the low incidence of tetanus in this age group. Just prior to the era of widespread vaccination, there were approximately 500 cases of tetanus each year.

To summarize this data, young people do not tend to get tetanus, and fatalities are extremely rare. Older people get tetanus more, and the case-fatality rate is higher (about 30 percent). Less than 100 cases of tetanus each year is a very low incidence, especially if a large percentage of the older population has no immunity. Tetanus has been almost completely eliminated from the United States, primarily because of good hygiene and proper wound management. Unlike the contagious diseases, the use of vaccines in some of the population will not help to protect those who are not vaccinated.

Vaccine administration

The primary series of tetanus toxoid vaccination consists of four injections. The first three doses are given at two-month intervals (though the intervals may be longer without forfeiting immunity) and the fourth dose about one year after the third dose. Boosters are recommended at five years old and every ten years thereafter. If a child has had the initial series of shots and recommended boosters, he or she does not need any further shots after injuries. Tetanus toxoid is often combined with other vaccines (e.g., diphtheria and pertussis in DT and DTP), though it can be given alone.

Protection from tetanus following adequate vaccination lasts for at least twelve years. In people who have had at least two doses of tetanus toxoid at any time in their lives, response to a booster injection of toxoid is rapid and adequate to prevent tetanus if given within 72 hours after an injury.

For individuals who have had less than two previous injections of tetanus toxoid, an injection of Tetanus Immune Globulin, Human (TIG) is administered for serious wounds. This vaccine introduces antibodies directly into the body to fight tetanus bacteria. This process is known as passive immunization; the body does not develop its own antibodies. The antibody levels achieved with TIG are sufficient to protect against tetanus if the injection is given within 72 hours after the injury. For individuals who have previously received two or more tetanus toxoid injections at any time in their lives, a single booster dose of toxoid will produce enough antibody response to prevent tetanus if the booster is given within 72 hours after an injury.

Vaccine efficacy

There is no question that a series of tetanus toxoid injections is highly effective at preventing tetanus (Edsall, 1959). This has been documented in several large studies during World War II, and with studies of large groups of horses. The fact that nearly all recent tetanus cases in the United States occurred in individuals who had not received the recommended schedule of vaccinations provides further evidence that active immunization is extremely effective.

The effectiveness of Tetanus Immune Globulin (TIG) in protecting previously unvaccinated individuals at the time of injury is more difficult to document. It is not possible to conduct controlled studies in humans. Judging the efficacy of tetanus immune globulin in the prevention of tetanus must be accomplished by measuring antibody responses after injection and by clinical experience. TIG raises antibodies in previously non-immune individuals to levels that indicate adequate protection from tetanus for at least 28 days (McComb & Dwyer, 1963). In addition, the record of tetanus immune globulin in the prevention of fatalities from tetanus is also extremely good. Clinical experience with TIG has led to a high level of confidence in the immune globulin's ability to prevent tetanus and death from tetanus when used in adequate doses within the prescribed interval following injury. There have been rare cases of fatalities in individuals who received tetanus immune globulin soon after injury (Johnson, 1969), but it is generally assumed that one dose of TIG will provide protection from tetanus when administered soon after an injury.

Vaccine reactions

Tetanus toxoid is generally considered safe, yet even this vaccine causes occasional severe reactions. It has been associated with an overall reaction incidence of 3 to 13 percent (White, W.G. *et al.,* 1983; Relihan, 1969). Most adverse reactions include swelling and abscesses at the injection site (Church & Richards, 1985) or mild fever and illness, however severe allergic and nervous system reactions have been reported. Two **deaths** following tetanus injections given alone were reported, one in 1933 (Regamey, 1965) and one in 1973 (Staak & Wirth, 1973). These were attributed to **anaphylactic reactions**, severe systemic allergic responses resulting in shock and collapse within four hours of injection. Thirteen cases of life-threatening allergic reactions meeting this definition have been reported in the literature (Institute of Medicine, 1994). Since tetanus toxoid is frequently administered in combination with diphtheria toxoid to both children and adults, adverse reactions to the two vaccines become difficult to distinguish in modern practice.

Many cases of **central nervous system disease** following tetanus toxoid injection have been reported in the medical literature. These cases include demyelinating diseases, Guillain-Barré syndrome (a demyelinating inflammatory disease of the peripheral nervous system with rapid onset of motor weakness and loss of sensation), neuropathies, and encephalopathies. They are often accompanied by severe, debilitating symptoms and hospitalization. A few of these cases are summarized below.

- A 50-year-old man received a dose of tetanus toxoid after suffering a wound to his foot. Ten days later he developed muscle aching, lethargy, fatigue and headache. Two days after that he was admitted to the hospital with flaccid paralysis of the legs, no reflexes, loss of sensation, back pain, and inability to urinate. One month later his symptoms remained unchanged (Read *et al.*, 1992).
- An 11-year-old girl received a routine tetanus booster dose and three days later developed blindness in the right eye and light perception only in the left eye. Her optic discs were swollen on exam. Two days later she had partial paralysis of her legs and loss of bladder control, then more widespread sensory loss including a lack of vibrational and positional senses. Seven weeks later she still had some vision loss and decreased muscle power. Within one year she recovered (Topaloglu *et al.*, 1992).
- A 21-year-old man developed coma on two separate occasions (2.5 years apart) within eight days of tetanus toxoid injections (Schwarz *et al.*, 1988).
- A 36-year-old woman developed lethargy, slurred speech, and decreased sensation five days after receiving a tetanus booster. She recovered over the next year (Schlenska, 1977).
- A 42-year-old man received tetanus toxoid on three separate occasions over a period of 13 years. Following each vaccination he developed acute polyneuropathy diagnosed as Guillain-Barré syndrome (Pollard & Selby, 1978). A nerve biopsy revealed demyelination. Following his last injection he continued to experience multiple recurrences, and continued to show sensory findings on examination as of 1993 (Pollard, 1993).

Arthritis, or joint inflammation and swelling, has occurred following both tetanus toxoid given alone and in combination with diphtheria toxoid. For example, a 34-year-old woman received two doses of tetanus toxoid one month apart, and one week after the second dose she developed persistent inflammation in several joints. Laboratory tests confirmed that her condition was rheumatoid arthritis, a chronic and usually permanent disease (Jawad & Scott, 1989). In a review of 100 million doses of tetanus toxoid given over 15 years in Germany, 13 cases of "swelling and inflammatory changes of joints" were reported (Korger *et al.,* 1986). Ninety-nine cases of joint inflammation following tetanus and diphtheria vaccine (Td) were reported to the Monitoring System of Adverse Events Following Immunization (MSAEFI) operated by the CDC during the period 1979 to 1990. Of 39 patients available for follow-up, 12 had not recovered (Institute of Medicine, 1994).

The long-term adverse effects of tetanus toxoid are unknown.

Tetanus immune globulin (human) has not been associated with reactions. Since it is a product made from human serum, it may contain infectious material, though this possibility is highly unlikely. All globulin products are tested for contamination by known pathogens such as hepatitis and HIV viruses. The alcohol fractionation process used in the production of TIG is a further safeguard, since this processing destroys such contaminating microorganisms.

Tetanus Summary

1. Tetanus is a potentially life-threatening disease.
2. Infection occurs through wounds.
3. Incidence of tetanus is approximately 50 cases per year for the past 10 years; less than 10 of these cases are under 30 years old, and these cases are rarely fatal.
4. A series of tetanus toxoid injections does provide protection from tetanus for at least 10 years. Tetanus immune globulin protects unvaccinated individuals if they receive an injection soon after injury.
5. Immediate vaccine reactions are usually mild, though many severe reactions have been reported, some of them causing permanent disability and a few fatalities. Long-term adverse effects are unknown.

Recommendations

Parents need to decide whether the low risk from possible tetanus exposure warrants giving the vaccine. This is primarily an issue of parental comfort level and likelihood of exposure. A child who lives on a farm or works with horses is more likely to be exposed than one who lives in urban or suburban areas. Parental anxiety about tetanus may be high because the disease progresses rapidly and can attack healthy children. Each parent must make the difficult decision about the tetanus vaccine.

I cannot recommend the tetanus toxoid vaccine for most children because of the unknown risks from long-term effects of the vaccine. However, if a child has a high likelihood of exposure or is traveling to a foreign country where sanitation is poor and the incidence of tetanus is higher than the United States, then tetanus vaccine administration should be seriously considered.

Some tetanus vaccine issues are clear. There is no reason to vaccinate infants because they are extremely unlikely to injure themselves. Delaying the vaccine until children are older may prevent adverse effects. A child does not need any protection from tetanus until he or she is old enough to play outdoors and get scrapes and cuts. Children under two years old are not at risk of contracting tetanus.

Some parents may feel that the tetanus vaccine is necessary even if they have decided against giving other vaccines. Tetanus toxoid is available as a single vaccine, or combined with diphtheria toxoid, or combined with diphtheria and pertussis. Parents can therefore choose to give the tetanus vaccine alone. Do not allow your child to receive any vaccine you do not want.

Parents can decide to do one of two things:

1. Give the series of tetanus toxoid injections (preferably after 12 months of age). After the primary series, a child only needs boosters every 10 years, regardless of injuries sustained.
2. Avoid the routine series and give TIG (Tetanus Immune Globulin, human) only if a child has a serious wound or a deep puncture.

Anyone with a serious wound should receive tetanus immune globulin (TIG) if they have had less than two previous injections of tetanus toxoid. The human immune globulin (TIG) contains tetanus antibodies which will directly attack circulating tetanus bacteria. This will help prevent the multiplication of bacteria and developing infection if it is given within a few days of injury. TIG will not confer lasting immunity to tetanus. By contrast, tetanus toxoid will not provide adequate protection in previously unvaccinated people until the second dose of the series is given 1 to 2 months after the first. This is too long a period of time to protect a person from a wound that has already occurred.

All wounds should be adequately cleansed. This subject was discussed in an article by Drs. Skudder and McCarrol in the *Journal of the American Medical Association* in the 1960s, when physician encounters with unvaccinated people were more common than today. Their statements and recommendations help to establish guidelines for the treatment of wounds:

> Good wound care is probably the single most important factor in the prevention of tetanus in fresh wounds. This implies thorough cleansing of the wound and removal of all foreign bodies and devitalized [dead] tissue. This is important since the tetanus bacillus is an anaerobic organism and can grow only in necrotic tissue which has no blood supply.
>
> For adequate prophylaxis of tetanus, wounds must be divided arbitrarily into those considered tetanus prone and nonprone.... Any wound containing foreign material or devitalized tissue must be considered tetanus prone, as well as crushing injuries, deep second and third degree burns, [and] any infected wound....
>
> The severity of a wound is not a reliable guide to the likelihood of tetanus developing since the disease may arise from minor or even unnoticed injuries. Many tetanus prone wounds, however, can be converted to non-prone wounds by proper cleansing and debridement (Skudder & McCarroll, 1964).

Children who are not vaccinated should have all wounds carefully cleansed at home or by a qualified health professional. If a serious wound occurs, or if there is a question about the need for tetanus protection, then the advice of a qualified physician should be sought and the administration of tetanus immune globulin (TIG) should be considered.

Polio

A t its worst, poliomyelitis is a disease that invades the nervous system and produces weakness and flaccid paralysis of the muscles supplied by affected nerves. Polio has probably existed for centuries, but no major epidemics occurred until the end of the nineteenth century. During the period 1900–1930, 80 to 90 percent of those afflicted with diagnosed polio were under five years of age, and the disease received its name of "infantile paralysis." No epidemics have occurred in the United States since 1954.

In underdeveloped countries where sanitation is poor, polioviruses are widespread. Almost 100 percent of children develop antibodies due to infection in infancy. Paralytic cases are few, the great majority being minor illnesses, and epidemics are unknown. As standards of living change, epidemics can be predicted to occur within a few years. This may be due to lack of general exposure to the virus and subsequent greater susceptibility in large numbers of people when virulent strains appear later. Immunization campaigns have also been associated with dramatic increases in polio cases in developing countries.

The polio virus enters the body through the nose or mouth, and multiplies in the digestive tract. From there it can enter the bloodstream and may then infect nerve cells. Most cases (90 to 98 percent) of illness associated with poliovirus remain either inapparent or characterized by sore throat, headache, nausea, and abdominal pain. It is usually diagnosed as a cold or flu. Only one percent of infections results in paralytic disease. Only a small percentage of these cases have residual paralysis.

Paralytic polio begins with a minor illness followed by a few days of well-being. Then more severe symptoms occur with stiffness of the back and neck, and muscle pain. Paralysis of the arms and/or legs soon follows. Rarely, paralysis of the muscles of respiration occurs. Return of muscle power begins after a period of days or weeks, and usually reaches its limit in 18 months. After that, any residual paralysis is permanent. Fatalities occur in 5 to 10 percent of the cases of paralytic polio, usually from respiratory paralysis.

There is no effective specific orthodox treatment for paralytic polio. Homeopaths have treated cases of paralytic polio with reported success, though no studies of treatment effectiveness have been conducted.

Incidence

Wild polio does not exist in the United States or the Western Hemisphere at this time. One case of paralytic poliomyelitis was reported in Peru in 1991 (Centers for Disease Control, 1991a). Since that time the Americas have been polio-free. The goal of the World Health Organization since 1988 has been global eradication of polio by the year 2000 (Centers for Disease Control, 1994b). All cases of paralytic polio in this country since 1979 were either caused by the oral vaccine or contracted in a foreign country during travel. During the period 1980–1985, 55 cases of paralytic polio were reported. Of these cases, 51 were caused by the vaccine and 4 occurred in people returning from developing countries (Centers for Disease Control, 1986). An average of 8 cases of vaccine-associated paralytic poliomyelitis (VAPP) occur each year in the United States (Institute of Medicine, 1988). The risk of acquiring wild polio in the United States is zero.

Vaccine efficacy

Two forms of vaccine are available. The inactivated or killed-virus vaccine, IPV, is given by injection. It works by producing circulating antibodies only. Booster doses are required as antibody levels decline.

The oral live-virus vaccine, OPV (Sabin), produces both intestinal and circulating antibodies, which apparently persist at high levels for years. The oral live-virus vaccine (OPV) replaced the killed vaccine (IPV) in 1962. The oral vaccine was favored because it was easier to administer and had less adverse effects. It was expected to produce longer-lasting and more complete immunity, and to also produce immunity in unvaccinated contacts of vaccine recipients who spread the virus to others after vaccination.

Experience with the killed and live vaccines subsequent to that time has proven the contrary. Live vaccine actually causes paralytic polio. The killed vaccine works just as well, and killed vaccine is claimed to reduce the spread of naturally occurring viruses in the community (Salk & Drucker, 1988).

A great deal of controversy exists concerning the effectiveness of the polio vaccines. Proponents claim the vaccine was responsible for the dramatic decline in polio cases subsequent to the mass immunization campaigns of the late 1950s. Critics suggest that the epidemic just lost its steam. In Great Britain the incidence of death from polio was at its height in 1950. By 1956, when the vaccine campaign was begun, it had already declined by 82 percent. Walene James, in her book *Immunization: The Reality Behind the Myth,* accuses the medical profession of distorting statistics to prove the vaccine's efficacy.

Dr. Bernard Greenberg, a biostatistics expert, was chairman of the Committee on Evaluation and Standards of the American Public Health Association during the 1950s. He testified at a panel discussion that was used as evidence for the congressional hearings on polio vaccine in 1962. During these hearings he elaborated on the problems associated with polio statistics, and disputed claims for the vaccine's effectiveness. He attributed the dramatic decline in polio cases to a change in reporting practices by physicians. Fewer cases were identified as polio after the vaccination for very specific reasons. This discussion has relevance to other vaccine experiences as well, and his remarks are therefore quoted at length.

> Prior to 1954 any physician who reported paralytic poliomyelitis was doing his patient a service by way of subsidizing the cost of hospitalization and was being community-minded in reporting a communicable disease. The criterion of diagnosis at that time in most health departments

followed the World Health Organization definition: "Spinal paralytic poliomyelitis: signs and symptoms of nonparalytic poliomyelitis with the addition of partial or complete paralysis of one or more muscle groups, detected on two examinations at least 24 hours apart."

Note that "two examinations at least 24 hours apart" was all that was required. Laboratory confirmation and presence of residual paralysis was not required. In 1955 the criteria were changed to conform more closely to the definition used in the 1954 field trials: residual paralysis was determined 10 to 20 days after onset of illness and again 50 to 70 days after onset....

This change in definition meant that in 1955 we started reporting a new disease, namely, paralytic poliomyelitis with a longer-lasting paralysis. Furthermore, diagnostic procedures have continued to be refined. Coxsackie virus infections and aseptic meningitis have been distinguished from paralytic poliomyelitis. Prior to 1954 large numbers of these cases undoubtedly were mislabeled as paralytic poliomyelitis. Thus, simply by changes in diagnostic criteria, the number of paralytic cases was predetermined to decrease in 1955–1957, whether or not any vaccine was used....

There is still another reason for the decrease in the reported paralytic poliomyelitis cases in 1955–57. As a result of the publicity given the Salk vaccine, the public questioned the possibility of a vaccinated child developing paralytic poliomyelitis. Whenever such an event occurred, every effort was made to ascertain whether or not the disease was truly paralytic poliomyelitis.... We have been conditioned today to screen out false positive cases in a way that was not even imagined prior to 1954.

As a result of these changes in both diagnosis and diagnostic methods, the rates of paralytic poliomyelitis plummeted from the early 1950s to a low in 1957 (Intensive Immunization Programs, Hearings, 1962; p. 96–97).

These factors called into question the claims for polio vaccine efficacy and the polio vaccine campaign in general. Nonetheless the polio vaccines, both OPV and IPV, have been attributed with the elimination of polio from many countries throughout the world, including the United States.

Despite the goals for global eradication of polio, outbreaks continue to occur in vaccinated populations. These outbreaks cast doubts on the claims for polio vaccine effectiveness. A widespread outbreak of type 1 polio occurred in Oman during 1988 and 1989. A total of 118 cases occurred, primarily in children younger than 2 years old, despite a universal vaccination program and full coverage (at least 3 doses of OPV) for 87 percent of children by the age of 12 months. The high rate of paralytic polio in this population means that thousands of fully vaccinated children became infected during the outbreak. More than 25 percent of fully vaccinated children may have been infected in the areas affected by the outbreak. The authors of the published report from the Centers for Disease Control question the effectiveness of existing polio vaccines and the present dosage schedules (Sutter *et al.*, 1991).

An even larger epidemic of 305 polio cases in 1 to 7-year-old children occurred in The Gambia, western Africa, in 1986, in a vaccinated population. The effectiveness of three doses of OPV was only 72 percent in this population. In other African countries the presence of protective levels of polio antibodies after appropriate vaccination was correspondingly low—36 percent in Ghana, 48 percent in Nigeria, and 55–74 percent in Kenya. The authors of the Gambian polio epidemic study concluded, "protection was not achieved by a well-established vaccination program that had fully vaccinated an estimated 64 percent of the age group with the highest attack rate.... Therefore, we doubt that substantially higher efficacy will be achieved in other African countries using the same trivalent oral polio vaccine formulation and vaccination schedule" (Deming *et al.*, 1992).

In Taiwan an outbreak of 1,031 paralytic polio cases occurred in 1982, in a population with an 80 percent vaccination level of infants. Although the polio cases occurred predominantly in unvaccinated children, spread of polio in such high numbers implies that many thousands of children were infected. An interesting finding in this study was the attribution of polio cases to contaminated water sources. Children were 5 times more likely to contract polio if they received water from non-municipal rather than municipal sources (Kim-Farley *et al.*, 1984). This epidemic provides evidence that the level of sanitation rather than the vaccination level in a community contributes significantly to the incidence of paralytic polio.

Vaccine reactions

The oral live-virus polio vaccine (OPV) is capable of causing paralytic polio in the vaccine recipient and close contacts. The CDC case definition of **vaccine-associated paralytic poliomyelitis (VAPP)** includes the onset of disease symptoms within 7 to 30 days postvaccination, or the onset of disease in a contact of a vaccine recipient within 7 to 60 days. The attack rate of VAPP is much higher for individuals receiving their first dose of live vaccine compared to subsequent doses. The risk of acquiring polio from the oral live vaccine is estimated to be 1 case per 520,000 first doses distributed (Nkowane *et al.*, 1987). The risk to household contacts is estimated at about 1 per 6 million vaccinees, and 1 per 23 million for community contacts (Nightingale, 1977).

The statistics of VAPP frequency could be disputed because of the strict guidelines for the definition of vaccine-associated paralytic polio cases. VAPP may occur with greater frequency than vaccine researchers claim. For example, in a recent World Health Organization review of VAPP in Latin America, 33 percent of 6,000 cases of acute flaccid paralysis were eliminated from consideration as VAPP because it was not possible to determine the presence of neurologic sequelae 60 days after paralysis onset (Andrus *et al.*, 1995). These cases were apparently lost to follow-up. If a case was diagnosed as Guillain-Barré syndrome (GBS) or aseptic meningitis it was also eliminated from consideration, even though these symptoms could have been caused by the vaccine also. Of the 125 cases of acute flaccid paralysis that met the criterion of onset of symptoms within 4 to 40 days postvaccine and persistent documented paralysis longer than 60 days, 65 percent of the cases were eliminated from the final statistics because they were labeled GBS or meningitis. These kinds of statistical trimming procedures are notorious for reducing the apparent adverse effects reported for vaccines.

In Romania the incidence of VAPP in infants was found to be exceedingly high compared to other countries. For the period 1984 to 1992, the risk of VAPP following receipt of the first dose of oral vaccine was 1 case per 85,000 doses distributed (Strebel *et al.*, 1994) compared to 1:520,000 in the United States. The authors also concluded that the true level of risk could be even higher because they did not adjust for wastage of vaccine. A follow-up study suggested that the higher rate of VAPP reactions in Romania could have been caused by the frequency of intramuscular injections of other drugs such as antibiotics in vaccine recipients in that country compared to other nations (Strebel, 1995). This ability of injections to provoke paralytic polio had previously been noted for wild-type polio as well. An injection given during the incubation period of wild-type poliovirus in infected persons may increase the risk of paralytic disease (Wyatt, 1985; Sutter *et al.*, 1992).

Guillain-Barré syndrome (GBS), characterized by progressive muscle weakness and destruction of the myelin sheath of nerves, is a well recognized adverse effect of oral polio vaccine. A mass polio vaccination campaign in Finland during February and March, 1985 resulted in a higher incidence of GBS cases in the first two quarters of 1985 (16 total cases) compared to a mean incidence of GBS in the population of 3 cases per quarter during a six year surveillance period, 1981–1986. Ten of these cases (ages 15 to 73 years) were diagnosed with GBS within 10 weeks after vaccination with OPV (Kinnunen *et al.*, 1989). A second research group in Finland identified a cluster of 10 GBS cases in children ages 0.4 to 14 years old during 1985. This cluster of GBS cases also coincided with the OPV vaccine campaign (Uhari *et al.*, 1989).

The Vaccine Safety Committee has acknowledged that OPV causes both paralytic polio and Guillain-Barré syndrome (Institute of Medicine, 1994).

Oral polio vaccine contains live viruses grown in monkey kidney cell cultures. The possibility of vaccine contamination and **transmission of monkey viruses** through the vaccine has been a cause of grave concern. A virus harbored by monkeys could grow in the vaccine culture and infect a human receiving the live virus vaccine. In the early days of polio vaccine research, everyone assumed that monkey viruses caused no problems in humans. These viruses were not considered harmful to humans, and regulations of the 1950s referred only to the exclusion of "viable" microbial agents, not monkey viruses (Papers, 1959). However, monkey B viruses, first identified by Albert Sabin, the inventor of the oral polio vaccine, were shown to infect humans and to cause illness and death.

Since that time, many different monkey viruses have been

transmitted from monkeys to humans. One particular monkey virus, SV-40 (Simian virus 40), contaminated the IPV vaccine during the period 1954 to 1963. An estimated 10 million to 30 million Americans were exposed to SV-40 through IPV injections and hundreds of millions of people world-wide received the contaminated vaccine (Shah & Nathanson, 1976). Prior to 1961, vaccine manufacturers did not give monkeys a blood test for SV-40 before using their kidneys for vaccine production. No one knows whether the contaminated vaccine caused any form of illness or symptoms because adverse effects of the vaccine were never studied comprehensively. However, an increased incidence of brain tumors was found among persons who had received the contaminated vaccine (Geissler, 1990). A study of more than 58,000 women who had received IPV during the years that SV-40 contaminated the vaccine (1959–1965) showed a thirteenfold increased risk of brain tumors in their children (Rosa *et al.*, 1988). Because antibodies to SV-40 were not found in the mothers' blood, the authors concluded that the cancers were probably caused by an unidentified infection from the polio vaccine since they knew that the vaccine was contaminated with numerous simian viruses (Rosa *et al.*, 1988a). The SV-40 virus does cause problems in humans. It has been identified in human brain tumors, and associated with other cancers as well (Kyle, 1992).

In 1980, Robert Gallo of the National Cancer Institute identified the first retroviruses that infected humans, the two human T-lymphotropic viruses, HTLV-I and HTLV-II. These viruses cause leukemia and cancer of lymph nodes in people. Two years later a virus with remarkably similar effects was discovered in monkeys, designated the simian T-lymphotropic virus, STLV. In a search for the origins of HTLV in humans, researchers began looking for monkeys in the wild that harbored the STLV virus. Genetic studies of monkey STLVs showed that human HTLV was closely related to the simian virus seen in the African green monkey (Kanki *et al.*, 1985). Gallo proposed that HTLV originated in Africa, infecting humans and primates and was spread to the Americas by the slave trade.

A similar search for a monkey virus related to HIV (the human immunodeficiency virus) began in 1984. At this time the human AIDS-related virus was called HTLV-III, and later renamed HIV. A new virus was soon discovered in monkeys that caused simian acquired immune deficiency, simian AIDS. Researchers who isolated this virus named it SIV. Genetic studies have shown that SIV is approximately 50 percent related to HIV (Essex & Kanki, 1988).

Later studies of high risk populations in West Africa revealed that 10 percent of their blood samples had antibodies that reacted with both HIV and SIV. This West African virus was found to be more closely related to SIV than to HIV, and it was named HTLV-IV and later renamed HIV-2. The reactions of the human blood samples were indistinguishable from the antibody reactions of infected African green monkeys. According to retrovirus researcher Robert Gallo, SIV is "virtually indistinguishable from some human variants of HIV-2" associated with West African AIDS (Curtis, 1992). According to viral researchers, "people infected with HIV-2 have antibodies entirely cross-reactive with SIV antigens; in fact, it is impossible to distinguish between SIV and HIV-2 on the basis of serological criteria." They go on to confirm, "All of this suggests at least that the primate and human viruses share evolutionary roots and at most that there may have been interspecies infection—that SIV-infected monkeys transmitted the virus to humans or vice versa" (Essex & Kanki, 1988).

Later researchers also proposed that HIV-2 was probably spread to humans from the SIV-infected monkeys through scratches, bites, or blood exposures while humans hunted and butchered the West African mangabey monkeys in the wild (Nowak, 1992). Another simian virus, this time SIV from chimpanzees, proved to be remarkably similar to several HIV-1 viral strains, thus connecting AIDS in both the United States (HIV-1) and Africa (HIV-2) with primates (Huet *et al.*, 1990). Some researchers referred to this connection between SIV in chimpanzees with HIV as the missing link to the origins of HIV-1 in humans (Desrosiers, 1990). Similarly, HIV can infect macaque (Agy *et al.*, 1992) and African green monkeys (Lecatsas & Alexander, 1992). Researchers continually discover these connecting links between SIV and HIV strains, HIV in monkeys, and SIV infections in humans. SIV was found in the cancer cells of an AIDS patient (Bohannon *et al.*, 1991), and SIV infections have been discovered in laboratory workers, agricultural workers, and urban dwellers (Khabbaz *et al.*, 1992; Gao *et al.*, 1992).

Although the SIV virus causes AIDS in captive macaque monkeys, infected African green monkeys remain symptom-free.

Researchers found that a surprisingly high number of African green monkeys carried the SIV virus—30–70 percent of monkeys in the wild (Essex & Kanki, 1988). These were the same green monkeys used in polio vaccine production, and these carrier monkeys were never excluded from vaccine production because they appeared healthy. US government tests in 1976–1977 detected retroviruses in polio vaccines, but authorities approved them for release if the vaccine contained fewer than 100 organisms per dose (Kyle, 1992).

In 1976, however, researchers at the US Bureau of Biologics recorded that three samples of Lederle polio vaccine contained between 1,000 and 100,000 simian viruses per ml. of vaccine, a much higher concentration than later safety regulations allowed (Kyle, 1992). Vaccine manufacturers were so concerned about monkey virus contamination of live polio vaccines that some pharmaceutical companies (e.g., Merck and Co.) refused to participate in vaccine production (Developments ..., 1961).

Several investigators have speculated that the contamination of oral polio vaccine with monkey viruses may have been the origin of AIDS. They have criticized the "cut hunter" hypothesis in which African hunters were supposedly infected by contaminated monkey blood as taking too long to spread AIDS compared to the rapid epidemic that actually occurred. They have searched for a more massive population exposure of humans to infected monkeys. What better way to spread a lethal virus and ignite mass epidemics than giving live monkey viruses to humans in a vaccine campaign?

Such a massive vaccine campaign in the Belgian Congo (now Zaire, Rwanda, and Burundi) using an oral polio vaccine contaminated with monkey SIV virus may have started AIDS outbreaks in Africa (Elswood & Stricker, 1993; Curtis, 1992). An experimental oral polio vaccine campaign during 1957 to 1959 included 320,000 infants and children in that area of Africa, which then became the center of the radiating African AIDS epidemics. That vaccine was prepared in monkey kidney cells that were known to be contaminated with at least 18 different simian viruses (Hayflick *et al.*, 1962). The polio vaccine used in the Congo experiments was never approved for human use and never used after 1960 (Elswood & Stricker, 1994). This connection between the contaminated polio vaccine, the Congo polio experiments, and the first outbreaks of AIDS in Africa has led several independent investigators to suspect the vaccine as the origin of

AIDS (Pascal, 1991). One reviewer stated it boldly and simply: "It is difficult to believe that the outbreak of HIV infection in Africa at the same time and location as this mass polio vaccine trial is a coincidence" (Elswood & Stricker, 1994). On the weight of this evidence, a lawsuit was filed in 1994 in federal court on behalf of a 12-year-old girl who allegedly contracted AIDS in 1992 from a series of oral polio vaccines she received in 1982.

Oral polio vaccine was used in repeated monthly doses beginning in 1974 to treat recurrent genital herpes (Tager, 1974). This treatment could have seeded the homosexual population with these simian retroviruses, producing the first United States AIDS epidemics (Kyle, 1992).

Investigators called for the testing of polio vaccines for the presence of simian viruses (SIV). A panel was convened to assess the credibility of the polio vaccine hypothesis as the origin of AIDS. The Wistar Institute, producers of the polio vaccine used in the Congo experiments, financed this in response to accusations about contaminated vaccines. Not surprisingly, this panel found the argument that AIDS arose from the polio vaccine extremely unlikely: "The panel found flaws in every step of the hypothetical pathway of transmission. It points out that neither SIV nor HIV is known to infect or multiply in... cells from monkey kidneys."

They acknowledged that cell cultures could contain white blood cells infected with HIV, but they argued that the freezing and thawing cycles would have "greatly reduced concentration and infectivity of any contaminating retrovirus" (Poliovaccine, 1992). They neglected to explain, however, how the live polio vaccine could survive processing that destroyed other viruses. As a matter of fact, it could not. According to Tom Folkes, chief virologist of the retrovirus laboratory at the Centers for Disease Control, vaccine manufacturers could not kill one virus and have other viruses survive. He said in reference to the oral polio vaccine, "the fact that it's a live vaccine would indicate that they had not gone through any inactivation procedures to denature the AIDS virus, because it would probably denature the polio virus. So the polio virus is kept alive, and the SIV virus would just travel with it. The theory, the possibility is real" (Curtis, 1992). Finally, the panel could not refute the possibility of transmission, and suggested that relevant samples of vaccine stock be tested for HIV/SIV viruses (Poliovaccine, 1992).

This is exactly what a group of researchers at the National Institute for Biological Standards in England proceeded to do. They conducted a laboratory examination of oral polio vaccine preparations from 4 manufacturers used between 1975 and 1984, the era prior to testing for SIV contamination. They found no evidence of HIV or SIV gene sequences in these samples—but these were not the same cultures as those used in the period 1957 to 1960 in the Congo. A vaccine used 20 years later, in 1975, would not necessarily have the same problems of contamination as those used in the African vaccine campaign. They tested the wrong vaccines.

These researchers also studied the ability of monkey kidney cell cultures to grow HIV. Cell cultures from uninfected monkeys failed to support the growth of HIV when it was added to the culture. They claimed that HIV could not survive and multiply in the conditions required for the growth of poliovirus.

They conducted a third experiment as well. They infected monkeys with SIV, and examined cells derived from their kidneys. No SIV virus or SIV antigens could be found in the kidney cell cultures after 10 days. As a result of those studies the authors concluded that "there is no evidence for HIV or SIV contamination in the poliovaccines we examined and that SIV from infected monkeys would be unlikely to survive the procedures involved in the production of [vaccine] or to replicate under the conditions required for the growth of poliovirus" (Garrett *et al.*, 1993). However, they did not examine specimens of vaccine used in the original African experiments, nor did they prove that SIV could not contaminate the vaccine.

Until HIV is found in polio vaccine, the theories about transmission of AIDS from monkeys to humans through the vaccine will remain speculative. A new discovery has created another link between monkey viruses, polio vaccine, and mysterious debilitating illnesses. This time the detection of a virus in patients with chronic fatigue syndrome (CFS) led to the monkey again.

An unusual virus was isolated from at least two patients with CFS, a cytomegalovirus-like stealth virus. Comparison of DNA sequences with other known viruses showed that this stealth virus was closely related to a strain of simian cytomegalovirus found in African green monkeys (Martin *et al.*, 1995). The most likely source for infection by an African green monkey virus is the live polio vaccine. This study provides further evidence that the polio vaccine could harbor unrecognized simian viruses capable of causing chronic infections in humans. Dr. John Martin, professor of pathology at the University of Southern California and chief author of that study, called on the FDA and CDC to monitor the current live vaccine for this virus in order to prevent further exposure of children, the unwitting live vaccine recipients (Schwartz, 1995).

Viruses can only be detected in vaccines if researchers know what they are trying to find. Monkey viruses have been transferred from monkeys to humans through the live polio vaccine because manufacturers did not know about their existence. It is possible that still other unidentified monkey viruses that cause disease in humans could be contained in today's oral polio vaccine, their discovery awaiting further research findings. Infants exposed to these monkey viruses could develop infections transmitted from monkeys to humans, the same type of infections suspected in the spread of AIDS and chronic fatigue syndrome.

Killed or **inactivated polio vaccine (IPV)** has not been associated with significant adverse reactions. No reports of anaphylaxis have been reported (Institute of Medicine, 1994). A review of Guillain-Barré syndrome during the years 1949 to 1966 revealed five cases associated with IPV, but few details were described (Leneman, 1966). In 1955 a preparation of IPV produced by Cutter Biological contained active virus that caused 260 cases of poliomyelitis in vaccine recipients (Nathanson & Langmuir, 1963). It was determined that bottles of tissue culture fluid containing the virus had been stored prior to inactivation with formaldehyde and tissues that settled to the bottom of containers protected the virus particles from the formaldehyde treatment (Klein, 1972). Since the introduction of new manufacturing safety requirements stimulated by the Cutter incident, no similar cases have been reported.

Polio Summary

1. No cases of wild polio have occurred in the United States since 1979. The risk of a child acquiring polio in the United States is zero, except from the vaccine itself.
2. The vaccines have questionable effectiveness.
3. Oral, live-virus vaccine (OPV) does cause polio in vaccine recipients and contacts. It has caused Guillain-Barré syndrome (GBS) in recipients. It also may contain live monkey viruses that have been associated with human diseases.
4. Killed polio vaccine (IPV) may have some adverse effects, but does not cause polio in recipients.

Recommendations

Since the risk of acquiring polio is near zero if a child is not vaccinated, it seems unjustifiable to risk contracting polio or other diseases transmitted by monkey viruses from the live vaccine. The only likely means of exposure to polio are travel to a foreign country, and contact with the feces of another child who has been vaccinated with the oral vaccine within the previous 6 to 8 weeks. The latter exposure can be minimized by informing day care providers of the unvaccinated status of your child, and ensuring that they take proper precautions with handwashing and disposal of soiled diapers of recently vaccinated children.

If you still have concerns about polio, then the killed vaccine (IPV) is an option. This vaccine is used routinely by several nations throughout the world as the only preventive for polio. The recent development of an enhanced-potency inactivated polio vaccine (E-IPV) has overcome some of the problems associated with the lower effectiveness of the old vaccine and can be used in fewer doses. The 1988 Institute of Medicine panel on polio vaccine concluded:

> Most parents concerned only for their child's welfare and informed about the nature of the alternatives would be likely to prefer one of the IPV vaccination strategies.... [A vaccination schedule] in which two or more doses of E-IPV were given prior to OPV would reduce or even eliminate cases of

vaccine-associated paralysis in recipients of OPV and in their contacts (Institute of Medicine, 1988).

Vaccine authorities suggest that the oral vaccine is still needed to produce intestinal immunity and prevent the spread of polio virus if it is introduced into a community. Authorities suggest two or more doses of E-IPV followed by OPV at 18 months of age and at entry to elementary school (Institute of Medicine, 1988). This schedule would reduce the risk of acquiring polio from the oral vaccine from 1 in 560,000 to 1 in 10.5 million (Marcuse, 1989). In October, 1995 the CDC Advisory Committee on Immunization Practices voted to develop new recommendations for polio vaccination based on a sequential schedule of inactivated polio vaccine followed by oral polio vaccine (Lockett, 1995). However, a schedule of the killed vaccine can be used alone if parents choose to vaccinate against polio.

Pertussis
(Whooping cough)

The vaccine controversy has reached its emotional and political zenith with the publicity generated by pertussis vaccine reactions. Public awareness was fueled by media presentations that focused on deaths and nervous system damage suffered by children after pertussis vaccination. The media attention to this issue included television documentaries, books in the popular press (Coulter & Fisher, 1991), and many magazine articles. Children in countries throughout Europe and the United Kingdom no longer receive the pertussis vaccine. Japan has postponed pertussis vaccination until children are two years old. The United States Congress passed the National Childhood Vaccine Injury Act to provide compensation to parents of children injured by vaccines, all in response to this public scrutiny of vaccine reactions.

This heightened interest in the pertussis vaccine was stimulated by consistent reports of dramatic vaccine reactions and permanent damage suffered by children after vaccination. Reactions to the vaccine have included fever, persistent crying, encephalitis, epilepsy, retardation, and death. Other neurologic diseases have been associated with the vaccine as well.

Pertussis is an infectious disease of childhood, associated with a specific bacteria. It can have dramatic and alarming symptoms. The illness usually begins as a mild cold, which lasts for a week. Then the characteristic cough starts, which makes this disease recognizable,

especially when it occurs in children. The cough comes in paroxysms and is often preceded by a feeling of apprehension or anxiety
and tightness in the chest. The cough itself consists of short explosive expirations in rapid succession followed by a long crowing inspi-
ration. During the coughing spell, the child's face may become red
or even blue; the eyes bulge, and the tongue protrudes. A number of
such paroxysms are sometimes followed by spitting up a mucus plug
and vomiting. This will end the attack, and the child will rest. Many
of these attacks may occur in one day, more frequently at night and
in a stuffy room. They may be brought on by physical exertion, crying, and often by eating or drinking. Infants, and even older children, do not always have "whooping" with their cough, and in adults
the cough may be mild and never diagnosed at all. The disease usually lasts for at least 6 weeks regardless of treatment. Complications
of pertussis may include cerebral hemorrhage, convulsions and brain
damage, pneumonia, emphysema, or a collapsed lung. Deaths are
usually due to complicating respiratory infections. Pneumonia is the
most frequent cause of death in children under three years of age,
but fatalities in children over 12 months are rare.

Standard treatment with antibiotics may help reduce the period
of contagion to others and prevent complications. It does not change
the course of symptoms. Homeopathic treatment has been used
extensively in the past, and one recent study suggests there may be
a beneficial effect from homeopathy in pertussis cases (English,
1987b). This survey followed children who received a homeopathic
preventive for pertussis, who subsequently did contract the disease
and were then treated homeopathically. The results of this survey
suggest that the group of children treated with homeopathy experienced relatively mild cases of pertussis, compared to children who
received antibiotic treatment. The author of this study acknowledges
that the number of children followed was too small to make any
definitive conclusions about the efficacy of homeopathy in the treatment of pertussis.

Incidence

Pertussis still occurs with regularity as a common childhood disease.
Prior to 1940, it was estimated that 95 percent of all individuals had

some form of pertussis during their life. The incidence of pertussis has declined from at least 100 reported cases per 100,000 population during the period 1930–1945 to an average of 1.5 per 100,000 population during 1984–1993. Several thousand cases occur per year, most during childhood. During the 10 year period 1982–1991, an average of 5 reported deaths per year were associated with pertussis.

Pertussis has become an increasingly common cause of cough in adolescents and adults. Immunity derived from the vaccine wanes after 5 to 10 years (Bass, 1985), and pertussis vaccine cannot be administered past 7 years of age because of severe reactions. Pertussis occurs regularly in older children and adults who have been fully vaccinated (Cherry *et al.*, 1989).

An outbreak that occurred in a middle school is typical. Thirteen eighth-grade students had culture-confirmed pertussis despite full vaccination (Mink *et al.*, 1994). In an evaluation of college students with prolonged cough, 26 percent proved to have pertussis (Morgan *et al.*, 1992). Pertussis is now a typical disease of adults who did not develop permanent immunity from the disease in childhood.

Vaccine efficacy

The most reliable studies of vaccine efficacy involve vaccinated children living in a house with someone who has contracted the disease. These studies have shown a variation in vaccine efficacy of 63 to 91 percent (Cherry *et al.*, 1988). One study showed an efficacy of 80 percent 3 years after the last dose, 50 percent between 4 and 7 years, and none after 12 years (Lambert, 1965). This is not a very high level of efficacy. In other words, the vaccine may not work in a large percentage of children.

Vaccine reactions

The political cover-up, distortion of facts, and outright disinformation campaign of the vaccine industry has been well documented in the works of Coulter and Fisher (1991) and Miller (1996). Efforts to vindicate the pertussis vaccine have appeared in countless forms despite the many reports and studies documenting its toxicity. These reports have included official statements to the media, analysis and re-analysis of data, editorials denouncing vaccine critics, and denial in the face of incontrovertible facts.

Insistence on enormous controlled studies diverts attention from the legion reports of damaged children. This argument also allows vaccine researchers to continue to ignore parents whose lives have been tragically reversed by the sudden devastation caused by vaccines. This tactic of denial has been staunchly followed despite the overwhelming evidence mounted against the pertussis vaccine which contains pertussis toxin, "one of the most reactive substances in nature" (Coulter & Fisher, 1991).

Several large studies have been conducted to investigate pertussis vaccine adverse reactions because of the consistent publicity generated by case reports of severe reactions since the vaccine was introduced. Epidemiologists have difficulty attributing apparent reactions to the pertussis vaccine for several reasons. The most problematic is that fevers, seizures, and sudden unexplained death (SIDS) all occur during the first year of life in the unvaccinated as well as the vaccinated. Since 95 percent of children in the United States are vaccinated, it is impossible to find an unvaccinated control group. This problem has been partially circumvented in studies that compare children vaccinated with DTP versus those vaccinated with only DT. Other studies compare the incidence of disease conditions in recently vaccinated children compared to the background incidence, but that group has also been vaccinated.

Comparing the incidence of seizure disorders in recently vaccinated children with a background incidence in similarly vaccinated children will distort and prejudice a study's findings. Comparing the adverse effects of one neurotoxic vaccine with another will only show that one is more dangerous; the low incidence in an unvaccinated population will never be determined. Another difficulty encountered in the evaluation of case reports of reactions in the medical literature is their inclusion of children who received diphtheria and tetanus accompanying the pertussis component, making it difficult to attribute adverse reactions to the pertussis vaccine alone.

The most comprehensive pertussis study was conducted in Los Angeles during 1978–1979, at UCLA (Cody et al., 1981). Children who received the DTP vaccine were compared to those who received the DT vaccine, and reactions that occurred during the first 48 hours after vaccine administration were recorded. The most serious criticism of the UCLA study and similar studies is that the vaccine may cause delayed reactions not apparent within the first two days. Delayed reactions are difficult to distinguish from the background occurrence of these problems. Dr. Harris Coulter, medical historian and author of two books on vaccine damage, has postulated that a wide array of neurologic problems can be attributed to these delayed or initially imperceptible reactions. In fact, he says, these represent an allergic encephalitis which is only diagnosed when effects are observed later in life:

> Severe neurologic sequelae may also occur after vaccination in the absence of an acute reaction. When the baby reacts to a DPT shot with "a slight fever and fussiness for a few days," this may be, and often is, a case of encephalitis which is quite capable of causing even quite severe long-term neurologic consequences.... Any researcher who ignores or rejects the possibility that vaccination can cause the most serious neurologic disorders in the absence of a marked acute reaction will have to find grounds for distinguishing post-vaccinal encephalitis from encephalitis due to other causes (Coulter, 1990).

The UCLA study data show that 50 percent of vaccinees developed fever, 34 percent irritability, 35 percent had crying episodes, and 40 percent had localized inflammation. The more significant major reactions included 3 percent of children who had persistent inconsolable crying and screaming, and 31 percent with excessive sleepiness (compared to 14 percent in the DT controls). The authors claimed that the occurrence of seizures could not be statistically verified because of the small numbers of children (16,536 vaccinations in the total study), although 1 in 1,750 doses of DTP caused seizures, or 1 in 333 children suffered seizures within 48 hours of vaccination.

A study with larger numbers also found a significant difference in seizure occurrence when 134,000 children receiving DTP were compared to 133,000 DT recipients. The relative risk of seizures after DTP compared to DT was 5.3 (Pollock & Morris, 1983). The authors of this study also attempted to minimize their findings, this time questioning whether these reactions were overreported by participating physicians because of the adverse publicity concerning the pertussis vaccine.

The occurrence of **encephalopathy** following pertussis vaccine has been reported in hundreds of cases and evaluated in several large studies. Encephalopathy is a vague term that one study defined as a spectrum of characteristics including "altered levels of consciousness, confusion, irritability, changes in behavior, screaming attacks, neck stiffness, convulsions, visual, auditory and speech disturbances, motor and sensory deficit" (Alderslade *et al.*, 1981). Convulsions are the most dramatic and often the most immediate of these symptoms, therefore seizures have been reported most frequently in the literature. An early report in 1948 described 15 cases of encephalopathy following pertussis vaccination at Children's Hospital in Boston. These cases consisted of fever, irritability, convulsions, and coma occurring within 12 hours of pertussis vaccination (Byers & Moll, 1948). Six of these children suffered from permanent cerebral palsy, 6 had seizures and mental retardation, and 2 died of pneumonia.

A later study reviewed 107 cases of neurologic illness occurring within 48 hours of pertussis vaccination (Berg, 1958). Fifty-nine cases of encephalopathy were reported in a study in 1974 from Germany. Seizures occurred in 39, and 11 had abnormal brain scans (Ehrengut, 1974). The same year, another study reported 36 cases of encephalopathy in London that occurred within 24 hours of pertussis vaccination. Most were accompanied by seizures (Kulenkampff *et al.*, 1974). A report of 72 infants who suffered severe adverse reactions was published in 1979. Thirteen of these infants died, and 59 had seizures, shock, persistent screaming, and other severe involvement of the nervous system (Hennessen & Quast, 1979).

Controversy surrounds the issue of **permanent neurologic damage** (injury to the brain and retardation) caused by pertussis vaccine reactions. The typical case involves an initial seizure after the vaccine's administration, followed by recurrent seizures after a few days or weeks. Then mental and motor retardation become apparent over the ensuing months (Cherry *et al.*, 1988). Other cases of neurologic symptoms may include hyperactivity and attention deficit disorder, learning disabilities, and behavior problems. The most reliable research conducted to investigate neurologic disorders after DTP vaccine was carried out in England, Wales, and Scotland during 1976–1979 in the National Childhood Encephalopathy Study (NCES) (Alderslade *et al.*, 1981). This case-control study sought to find a risk factor for vaccine reaction by examining all cases of neurologic disease, and comparing those cases to a control group. Only hospitalized cases were examined. DTP vaccination had occurred significantly more frequently within the previous 72-hour and seven-day periods in the children with neurologic illness than in the controls. The estimated risk of serious neurologic disorder within seven days after DTP was 1:110,000 vaccinations, and the estimated risk of persistent neurologic damage 1 year later was 1:310,000.

These figures have been assailed by parties on both sides of the controversy. Through an analysis of the data, Dr. James Cherry of UCLA and his colleagues determined that the temporal association of DTP with neurologic disease merely indicates that the vaccine had brought out symptoms that would have occurred anyway. The High Court of England declared that the NCES data and conclusions were premature and based on interim figures. The Court effectively reversed the findings of permanent neurologic damage based on follow-up findings of the cases in question (Bowie, 1990).

This assessment was reiterated in the medical reviews published in the United States as well: "We do not know whether pertussis vaccine causes permanent brain damage" (Wentz *et al.*, 1990). That review concludes that a study would need to include approximately 4,000,000 vaccinated children in order to reach some definitive conclusion about permanent neurologic damage caused by the vaccine. The prohibitive cost of such a study assures that it will never be conducted.

However, a follow-up study in 1993 of permanent neurologic damage suffered by the children in the NCES data confirmed that these children continued to display neurologic abnormalities, thus vindicating the original findings of this study. This study traced over 80 percent of the children who suffered severe acute neurological illness following pertussis vaccine, as well as control children. All surviving children were administered a battery of intelligence and achievement tests; questionnaires on behavior and progress were completed by parents and teachers; and clinical and neurologic exams were performed by physicians. The authors concluded that "Case children were significantly more likely than controls to have died or to have some form of educational, behavioural, neurological, or physical dysfunction a decade after their illness" (Miller *et al.*, 1993).

Two follow-up studies of 16 children with neurologic reactions in the UCLA study showed continuing abnormalities in those children as well. In the follow-up study sponsored by the FDA, 13 children were administered neurologic and educational examinations. These researchers found normal performance IQ scores (104.3 ± 15.8) and low verbal IQ scores (91.8 ± 18.4). One child had a verbal IQ score of 65 and performance IQ score of 88. Another had a verbal IQ score of 70 and performance IQ score of 106. The authors casually remark that "these lower verbal IQ scores can be explained by the proportion of Hispanic and bilingual children in this sample." If the researchers were not so eager to discount the findings of IQ scores in the mentally retarded range in these vaccine damaged children, perhaps they might have administered these tests in Spanish. Despite this overall discrepancy between performance and verbal IQ, a criterion for language processing disability, the authors conclude, "there is no evidence that any of these 16 children suffered any serious neurologic damage as a result of either convulsions or hypotonic-hyporesponsive episodes" (Baraff et al., 1988).

Evaluation of these same children by an independent pediatric neurologist who administered IQ tests in Spanish when necessary revealed significant language and learning disabilities in these children. These included significant discrepancies between verbal and performance IQ, as well as language delays, attention deficit disorder, motor abnormalities, borderline low IQ, and mental retardation. His conclusion about these same children was drastically different than the government sponsored findings. In reporting his evaluations to an Institute of Medicine Committee researching pertussis vaccine reactions, he stated, "Only 4 of the 13 tested were unequivocally normal" (Gabriel, 1990).

Given the controversies surrounding the association of permanent neurologic damage to pertussis vaccine in these two studies, the Institute of Medicine Committee found insufficient evidence to establish a causal relation between these permanent symptoms and the vaccine (Institute of Medicine, 1991).

Dr. Harris Coulter and his co-author, Barbara Loe Fisher, insist that the NCES and UCLA figures grossly underestimate the true extent of damage caused by the pertussis vaccine, because the criteria for timing of symptom occurrence are much too limited, and definitions of reactions are chosen to minimize findings (Coulter & Fisher, 1991). In fact, Coulter would attribute a much larger number of "soft" neurologic symptoms (learning disorders, attention deficits, and behavior problems) to the vaccine. He suggests that delayed vaccine reactions are often responsible for these permanent disabilities (Coulter, 1990). The fevers and sleepiness that occur frequently after pertussis vaccine represent an initial assault on the brain that results in permanent damage, disabilities, and abnormalities. These initial short-term reactions are just the tip of the iceberg, according to Coulter, that accounts for a wide range of behavioral problems in children and in adults including criminal behavior, homelessness, and drug abuse.

The relationship of pertussis vaccine to **deaths** is even more controversial. The reports of many deaths following DTP vaccination led investigators to conduct studies on the incidence of SIDS (sudden infant death syndrome) and its relationship to DTP. In 1979, 4 infants in Tennessee all died within 24 hours of their first DTP vaccination (Hutcheson 1979). All of these children received the same lot of vaccine. Two sets of twins, aged 5 and 10 months, died within 24 hours of DTP (Roberts, 1987; Werne & Garrow, 1946). And one study summarized case reports of more than 150 deaths following DTP by 37 authors in 12 countries (Torch, 1986).

Three studies have found a temporal association between infant deaths and DTP vaccination (Baraff *et al.*, 1983; Torch 1982; Walker *et al.*, 1987). In Walker's case-control study, the relative risk for SIDS (sudden infant death syndrome) within 3 days of vaccination was 7.3, a very significant risk (Walker, 1990). The Torch study found an increased incidence of SIDS in the period immediately after vaccination compared to a control period several weeks later. The Baraff study concluded, "The excess of deaths in the 24 hours and one week following immunization and the absence of deaths in the fourth week following immunization were all statistically significant."

At least 4 other studies found no significant association between SIDS and pertussis vaccination. Two of these studies included large populations of children, and they are most frequently cited as the best evidence that SIDS has no relationship to the vaccine. The largest study included an analysis of 716 cases of SIDS during the period 1978–1979 in a birth population of 350,000 children (Hoffman *et al.*, 1987).

The methods of this study have been assailed in a critique submitted to the Institute of Medicine (Coulter, 1990b). The conclusions of that critique discount the study's findings. "In fact, these results prove nothing at all, and this study is just an exercise in confusion.... As the study was done, no meaning can be extracted from it." The manipulation of data in that study clearly attempted to disprove the connection to SIDS, and study methods were biased to ensure that the finding of an association did not occur. The other major study cited as proof that SIDS is unrelated to pertussis vaccination is the notorious Griffin fiasco of 1988. That study's methods were discussed in Part I (page 15) where bias, lack of follow-up, and exclusion of significant findings were revealed as major flaws in this political attempt to exonerate the pertussis vaccine. Not unexpectedly, the American Academy of Pediatrics Task Force on Pertussis concluded that there is no convincing evidence for a causative role for DTP vaccination in SIDS in their review of these 7 studies (Cherry et al., 1988). The Institute of Medicine committee formed to review adverse consequences of pertussis vaccine reached the same conclusion (Institute of Medicine, 1991).

Anaphylaxis, sudden onset of a life-threatening allergic reaction and systemic collapse, has been recognized as a consequence of many vaccines including pertussis. In one report of DTP reactions, 7 infants had severe shock with loss of consciousness or swelling of the larynx (Osvath et al., 1979). Another study reported 8 children with anaphylaxis or collapse within 24 hours of DTP vaccination, for a rate of 6 cases per 100,000 children vaccinated (Pollock & Morris, 1983). Other individual cases of anaphylactic reactions have been reported as well (Leung, 1985; Ovens, 1986; Cody et al., 1981; Galazka et al., 1972).

Hemolytic anemia, the destruction of red blood cells that could be caused by toxic agents or antibody responses to vaccines (Facktor et al., 1973), has been associated with the DTP vaccine. One report cited 3 cases of hemolytic anemia in infants after DTP. These occurred in a 4-month-old boy 4 days after vaccination, a 6-month-old girl hospitalized with anemia 3 weeks after vaccination, and a boy aged 10 months who had been sick for weeks following his DTP vaccination at 6 months (Haneberg et al., 1978). Another case of acute hemolytic anemia following vaccination was discovered in a review of 44 children with autoimmune hemolytic anemia (Zupanska *et al.,* 1976). A 2.5-year-old boy developed hemolytic anemia six days after his fourth dose of DTP and then again 6 days after his fifth dose (Coulter & Fisher, 1991).

Regardless of these controversies, it is clear that the pertussis vaccine is dangerous. Parents must ultimately decide whether they want to risk reactions to vaccination. It is parents who are responsible for the passage of the vaccine compensation law. Parents initiated the lawsuits which have consistently resulted in monetary awards for vaccine damage, and the pertussis vaccine has been at the forefront of this controversy. Many countries have stopped the use of pertussis vaccines because of its associated risks.

Pertussis Summary

1. The vaccine is associated with severe reactions including encephalitis, seizures, brain damage, and deaths.
2. The disease itself has these same risks, though the incidence of pertussis is now low in the United States.
3. The vaccine has limited efficacy.
4. The disease can be treated with homeopathic medications.

Recommendations

I advise against the pertussis vaccine because of the significant risk from the shot, and because homeopathy is able to provide treatment for whooping cough when it occurs (English, 1987b). Before anyone gives their child a pertussis shot, I recommend that they read the case descriptions in Coulter and Fisher's book. No amount of controversial statistics can compare to the harrowing and heart-rending accounts of parents with vaccine-injured children.

Acellular Pertussis

The public outcry over the tragic adverse effects of the currently used whole-cell pertussis vaccine has spurred a search for safer vaccines. Drug manufacturers are being pressured to develop a vaccine with less severe reactions. This occurred in Japan, and to a lesser extent in the United States. In 1981, the Japanese switched from a whole-cell pertussis vaccine to a more complex acellular vaccine, primarily because of public pressure. Parents began refusing to give their children the whole-cell vaccine. The "improved" acellular vaccine was introduced to quell fears about the shots since the supposedly toxic components were removed.

The first acellular pertussis vaccine was licensed in the United States in 1991 for use as the fourth and fifth doses of the recommended DTP schedule for children ages 16 months through 6 years (Centers for Disease Control, 1992c). Japanese studies had shown that the acellular vaccine was 79 to 97 percent effective, depending on the definition of effectiveness, in children older than 2 years (Mortimer *et al.*, 1990). Acellular vaccine was adopted for use as a booster in older children, in an attempt to reduce severe reactions to the pertussis component of DTP in this age group.

Vaccine efficacy

Swedish studies have evaluated the effectiveness of acellular pertussis vaccines in the prevention of whooping cough. For culture-confirmed pertussis, the observed efficacy was 64 percent for one strain and 54 percent for another strain of acellular vaccine (Ad hoc group, 1988). Sweden withdrew an application for licensure of the vaccine on the basis of these tests (License, 1989).

Vaccine Reactions

This vaccine seems to cause fewer of the mild-type reactions than the older whole-cell vaccine. In Japan, the replacement of whole-cell with acellular vaccine resulted in a 60 percent reduction of "mild" reactions, particularly febrile seizures. But the rate of severe reactions did not differ significantly between the acellular and whole-cell vaccine (Noble *et al.*, 1987). Several small studies have evaluated the rates of mild and systemic reactions to various preparations of acellular vaccine in the United States in infants (Pichichero *et al.*, 1992) and older children between 17 months and 6 years of age (Halperin *et al.*, 1994; Bernstein *et al.*, 1992). The Japanese experience with acellular vaccine has included only children 24 months or older. There are no data that allow us to predict the rate of severe reactions for infants given the new vaccine (Cherry *et al.*, 1988).

A recent study in Sweden also revealed that the acellular vaccine caused less of the mild-type reactions than the whole-cell vaccine. But encephalitis reactions did occur with the acellular vaccine. A total of 212 infants received the acellular vaccine. Two serious reactions occurred. These reactions are identical to those following the whole-cell vaccine. The case descriptions are quoted here at length.

- A girl who had received two doses of the acellular vaccine as primary vaccination started to cry persistently 7 hours after the booster injection. The parents had never heard such a cry before. She cried for 1.5 to 2 hours, and then went to bed and slept normally. The following morning she was found in bed pale, hypotonic, and unresponsive.
- A boy who had received three doses of the acellular vaccine as primary vaccination became fretful and tired, and refused to eat 2 to 3 hours after the booster injection. The unusual behavior of the child continued, and he was hospitalized the following day. These symptoms recurred periodically during the 4

days of hospitalization. Clinical and laboratory examinations yielded no signs of infection or hypoglycemia. The boy recovered fully. Two EEGs [studies of brain waves] showed pathologic activity. The diagnosis was focal encephalitis of unknown origin (Blennow and Granstrom, 1989).

These limited studies of the acellular vaccine reveal that children vaccinated during infancy have serious vaccine reactions. In the Swedish study the rate of serious reactions was 1 in 100 vaccinated children. The limited scope of this study does not allow us to draw conclusions about frequency of severe reactions, but this rate is much *higher* than that reported for the current whole-cell vaccine.

Another Swedish study observed 2,800 infants who received acellular pertussis vaccine in a double blind placebo-controlled experiment with the vaccine. Four of the children died within 2 weeks to 5 months of vaccination. Their cases are summarized here.

- A previously healthy 10-month-old girl developed *H. influenzae* meningitis 9 days after her second dose of acellular pertussis vaccine and she was hospitalized that day. Five days later she died. Autopsy revealed severe brain damage.
- A 15-month-old boy began having symptoms 10 weeks after his second vaccination. He cried during the night, and then had convulsions at 4:00 AM. He was found dead 5 hours later.
- A third baby died of meningitis 5 months after his second dose of vaccine.
- The fourth baby, a 12-month-old girl was found dead in her bed 1 month after vaccination, but morphine was discovered in her blood and her death was probably from poisoning (Storsaeter *et al.,* 1988).

The reports of the two fatalities that were possibly related to the acellular pertussis vaccine contributed to the decision of Swedish authorities to recommend withdrawal of the application for vaccine licensure. They said, "The Division of Drugs judges that the efficacy of the vaccine may be lower than that of whole-cell vaccines. The uncertainty about a possible association with deaths due to serious bacterial infections, which occurred among vaccinated children, has also contributed to the recommendation" (License, 1989).

The pertussis vaccine is dangerous in all forms developed thus far. The Japanese experience with use of acellular vaccine beginning at 2 years of age shows that reactions are significantly reduced if vaccination is delayed, whether whole-cell vaccine or acellular vaccine is used. Infants will continue to be severely damaged by these pertussis vaccines, and the true extent of undetected, long-term disease may never be discovered.

Acellular Pertussis Vaccine Summary

1. Severe reactions to the whole-cell pertussis vaccine have spurred worldwide efforts to produce a safer vaccine.
2. The acellular form of the pertussis vaccine seems to diminish mild-type reactions compared to the whole-cell vaccine.
3. Severe reactions to the acellular vaccine also occur, including encephalitis and possibly death.

Diphtheria

Diphtheria is an acute infectious disease caused by a bacterium. The disease is characterized by a sore throat, and the development of a membrane that may cover the throat. It can become a dangerous disease if this membrane makes it difficult or impossible to breathe. Complications of diphtheria include (1) myocarditis (infection within the heart), which can lead to heart failure, and (2) transitory paralysis of the limbs, muscles of respiration (sometimes causing death), or muscles of the throat or eye. The incubation period is two to four days.

Incidence

Diphtheria is now an extremely rare disease in the United States. The number of cases has steadily declined during the past century. For example, between 1900 and 1920 the mortality rate from diphtheria declined by 50 percent, before the widespread use of diphtheria vaccine (Mortimer, 1978). The toxoid vaccine was invented in 1923 and came into widespread use over the next 15 years. Prior to that time, a toxin-antitoxin preparation had been used in more limited settings after its discovery in 1914. During the 1940s, reported diphtheria cases numbered 15,000 to 30,000 per year in the United States. By the 1960s the number of cases declined to 200 to 1,000 per year. And in the 1980s there were 0 to 5 cases per year.

Vaccine efficacy

There is some question about the effectiveness of diphtheria vaccine. A classic situation occurred in Germany during World War II. When diphtheria vaccination was made mandatory, there was a 17 percent increase in the number of cases and a 600 percent rise in the number of deaths from diphtheria. When the vaccine was stopped at the end of the war, the incidence of diphtheria dramatically declined, despite the poor living conditions and malnutrition. During an epidemic of diphtheria in Chicago during 1969, 25 percent of the cases had been fully vaccinated, and an additional 12 percent showed serologic evidence of full immunity, though they had received less than the full series of shots (Mendelsohn, 1978).

Vaccine reactions

Diphtheria toxoid is given only in combination with tetanus toxoid, and reactions are therefore impossible to attribute to one or the other vaccine. Reactions that do occur are usually attributed to tetanus because tetanus toxoid, when given alone, causes these reactions also. Early studies of diphtheria toxoid showed that vaccination caused severe local and systemic reactions (fever, muscle aches, fatigue, headaches, and chills). These problems were alleviated by improved manufacturing methods and reduction of the dose of vaccine (Edsall *et al.*, 1954; Myers *et al.*, 1982).

Diphtheria Summary

1. Diphtheria is a potentially serious disease, but extremely rare in the United States, with an incidence of less than 5 cases per year.
2. The vaccine has questionable effectiveness.
3. Long-term effects of the vaccine are unknown.

Recommendations

At the present time this vaccine seems unnecessary due to the low incidence of disease and questionable vaccine efficacy.

Measles, Mumps, and Rubella

Vaccination for these diseases is usually given as a single shot of combined live viruses (the MMR vaccine) at 12 months of age or older. Mass vaccination of children for mumps, measles, and rubella has resulted in a shift in the pattern of these diseases. The age distribution has changed significantly since the vaccines were introduced in the 1960s. Now these are increasingly becoming diseases of adolescents and young adults. This is a problem, since the diseases themselves cause more complications in this older population.

The vaccines seem to have caused atypical forms of the diseases to appear. It should also be remembered that the natural occurrence of each of these viral diseases generally confers permanent immunity against subsequent attacks.

Measles

Measles was a common disease of childhood prior to the widespread use of measles vaccine. The disease is transmitted by a virus that is highly contagious. The symptoms of measles are cold symptoms, cough, irritated eyes, and high fever, with the appearance of a rash on the fourth day of illness. The symptoms, including the rash, reach a climax on about the sixth day and then subside in a few days.

Measles occasionally sets the stage for other diseases. These complications include ear infections, pneumonia, infection of lymph nodes, and encephalitis, but they are not common. In the past, deaths from measles were not uncommon during epidemics. Now the disease has become milder and deaths are rare. Measles is usually a self-limited disease. Encephalitis is reported to occur in one out of 1,000 cases, though this figure is probably exaggerated. Of these encephalitis cases, 25 to 30 percent show manifestations of brain damage.

Orthodox medicine has no specific treatment for measles or measles-associated encephalitis. Homeopaths feel confident about their ability to prevent complications, though no efficacy studies have been conducted.

Incidence

Measles was contracted by most children prior to vaccine licensure. Following the licensing of measles vaccine in 1963, the incidence of measles declined to an average of 3,000 cases per year in the 1980s (Centers for Disease Control, 1994). However, in 1989, a resurgence of measles occurred in the United States, constituting an epidemic that brought levels back up to the 1970s rate of 27,000 reported cases per year. After that epidemic, reported cases declined again to the pre-epidemic levels.

This increase in measles cases came as a blow to the vaccine campaign promoters who had made claims to eliminate measles from the United States. This setback was a disappointment, because just prior to that epidemic vaccine proponents had been congratulating themselves that the incidence of reported measles had declined to less than 2 percent of previous levels (Markowitz et al., 1989). The 1982 date that had been set for the elimination of measles had passed, but researchers were hopeful and confident. They claimed that "epidemics no longer occur," and self-congratulatory statements were commonplace: "Because of the success of measles-control efforts in the United States, a goal of measles elimination has been established here and in other countries" (Markowitz et al., 1989). All of this success was attributed to the vaccine.

Then the epidemic of 1990 hit, primarily in preschool-age children. In fact, nearly 20 percent of measles cases in 1990 and 1991 occurred in children less than 1 year of age. What did researchers blame for this resurgence of cases in babies? The vaccine. "The cause of the increase in measles cases among children <15 months of age is ... earlier susceptibility to measles due to transplacental transfer of lesser amounts of measles antibody from young mothers whose measles immunity is from vaccine rather than wild measles virus" (Centers for Disease Control, 1992b). Mothers, in other words, who grew up in the measles vaccine era do not pass antibodies to their babies because immunity from the vaccine disappears over time. Now the shift has occurred from measles as a childhood disease to measles as a disease of adults—and infants born to these adults. Both groups tend to have more complications. The thirty year fiasco continues.

Vaccine efficacy

The vaccine has apparently resulted in a dramatic decline in measles cases. In the light of these promising statistics, a national goal was set to eliminate measles by 1982. Notwithstanding these hopes, reports of epidemics in fully vaccinated populations have appeared periodically and consistently since the vaccine's introduction (Shasby *et al.*, 1977; Weiner *et al.*, 1977; Hull *et al.*, 1985).

A typical example was reported by Dr. Tracy Gustafson and colleagues in the *New England Journal of Medicine*. During the spring of 1985, a measles outbreak occurred in two fully vaccinated secondary-school populations (greater than 99 percent of students vaccinated). On serologic testing, 95 percent of students showed immunity to measles. The epidemic occurred in the remaining 5 percent, all of whom had been "adequately" vaccinated (Gustafson *et al.*, 1987).

Some authors have postulated that a waning immunity over time is responsible for these outbreaks among older children (Shasby *et al.*, 1977). Others blame primary vaccine failure. In any case, the public health goal of eradicating measles in the United States by 1982 was not met, despite rigorous vaccine programs.

Gustafson concluded in 1987 that such a goal is impossible to meet. She was right. In an attempt to counteract the resurgence of measles, CDC announced a two-dose measles schedule (Centers for Disease Control, 1989i), but a new epidemic again foiled the goals for measles eradication. Nonetheless, a new date was set for elimination of measles in 1996 (Centers for Disease Control, 1994c). In frustration, other researchers also admitted that eradication of measles may not be possible since transmission continues to occur in adolescents and adults who have been fully vaccinated. Their understated and plaintive response was, "Measles elimination has proved more difficult than previously predicted" (Hersh *et al.,* 1991).

Measles cases now consistently occur in the vaccinated. A review of measles outbreaks in the United States during 1985–1986 revealed that a median of 60 percent of cases in school-age children occurred in vaccinated individuals (Markowitz *et al.,* 1989). Similarly, a review of 1,600 cases of measles in Quebec, Canada, between January and May, 1989 showed that 58 percent of school-age cases had been previously vaccinated (Centers for Disease Control, 1989a). In states with comprehensive (kindergarten through 12th-grade) immunization requirements, between 61 and 90 percent of measles cases occur in persons who were "appropriately" vaccinated (Markowitz *et al.,* 1989).

The official response to measles vaccine failure and epidemics has varied. Within the first ten years after widespread vaccination, the vaccine failures prompted public health authorities to repeatedly raise the recommended age for vaccination. In 1969, the age for vaccine administration was raised to 12 months or older (Albrecht *et al.,* 1977). Because of continued vaccine failure, the age for administration was subsequently raised to 15 months (Centers for Disease Control, 1989b). During 1988, an epidemic in Los Angeles prompted a reconsideration of vaccine recommendations when statistics showed that 38 percent of cases were less than 16 months old (Centers for Disease Control, 1989c). The age for vaccine administration was then lowered again to 9 months in areas with recurrent measles transmission (Centers for Disease Control, 1989d). These children would then require revaccination at 15 months.

The fact that a large percentage of measles cases occurs in school-age children and adolescents resulted in the recommendation of mass revaccination. The American College Health Association recommended that all colleges and universities require documentation of both measles and rubella immunity as a prerequisite to matriculation (ACHA, 1983). And finally, the Centers for Disease Control and American Academy of Pediatrics announced that the measles vaccine failures necessitated a second dose of vaccine (Centers for Disease Control, 1989i).

It is clear that chasing vaccine failure and establishing ambitious eradication goals has not produced the great successes promised.

Vaccine reactions

The list of adverse reactions associated with the measles vaccine is shamefully long. The measles vaccine has proven to be a failed and tragic experiment. Vaccine apologists assure us through statistics that natural measles would cause the same effects as vaccination, but in greater numbers. This is small compensation to parents of children who have been injured by the measles vaccine.

The problems caused by the measles vaccine read like a neurologic textbook. Encephalitis, meningitis, subacute sclerosing panencephalitis, seizure disorder, sensorineural deafness, optic neuritis, transverse myelitis, Guillain-Barré syndrome. The human tragedy described in the hundreds of reports is staggering. This vaccine is dangerous. Yet the final twist on this extravagant failure is that the Vaccine Safety Committee ignores their own findings and would have us believe that inadequate evidence exists to prove an association between vaccination and these devastating diseases. The only conditions attributed to the MMR vaccine are thrombocytopenia and anaphylaxis (Institute of Medicine, 1994). Such denial amounts to a travesty of adverse event reporting. Why report these events at all, if the vaccine industry chooses to ignore them?

The following descriptions of adverse reactions sometimes occurred following measles vaccination alone. When measles vaccine is administered in the combination MMR vaccination, attributing reactions to one vaccine is difficult unless specific antibody studies confirm the specific cause. Reactions to MMR vaccine are included in this chapter.

One of the most dangerous reactions caused by measles vaccine is an inflammatory response in the brain known as **subacute sclerosing panencephalitis (SSPE)**. This disease causes demyelination of nerve sheaths and a slow, progressive deteriorating condition, resulting in death, often within 1 to 2 years. Its association with natural measles infection is well-established.

The first reported case of SSPE following measles vaccine occurred in 1968, in a child with onset of symptoms within 3 weeks of vaccination. The child died 18 months later (Schneck, 1968). Within 5 years of that report, 22 additional cases of measles vaccine associated SSPE were reported in the medical literature (Jabbour *et al.,* 1972). In 1969, a registry was established to document cases of SSPE and its association to measles vaccine. The registry now includes data on more than 575 patients (Institute of Medicine, 1994). Although the annual incidence of SSPE has declined since the 1970s, accompanying the decline in natural measles, the proportion of cases with an antecedent history of measles vaccination has increased (Dyken *et al.,* 1989).

Reports of central nervous system disorders following measles vaccination abound throughout the worldwide medical literature. A review of cases reported to the Centers for Disease Control from 1963 to 1971 revealed 59 patients with extensive neurologic disorders (Landrigan & Witte, 1973). In the United Kingdom, 47 cases of encephalitis were reported between 1968 and 1974, and 122 febrile convulsions occurred following measles vaccinations (Beale, 1974). Another report from England identified 26 cases of convulsions between 1975 and 1981 after vaccination (Pollock & Morris, 1983). A report of adverse events associated with measles vaccine in Japan from 1978 to 1983 described 12 cases of encephalitis (Hirayama, 1983). Cases reported through VAERS included 17 suggestive of encephalopathy or encephalitis (Institute of Medicine, 1994).

Other neurologic problems have been seen following measles vaccination. **Guillain-Barré syndrome (GBS),** an autoimmune disease characterized by paralysis and demyelination of nerve sheaths, occurred in a 19-month-old girl after measles vaccine. Within 1 week following vaccination she was unable to stand. A second girl, aged 10 months, developed GBS within 4 days of measles, DTP, and OPV vaccination (Grose & Spigland, 1976). A 12-year-old girl was diagnosed with GBS following MMR vaccination (Norrby, 1984) and a total of 17 cases developed GBS following measles or MMR vaccination in the MSAEFI and VAERS reporting systems between 1979 and 1992 (Institute of Medicine, 1994). Cases continue to be reported. In 1994 a report appeared describing a 16-month-old girl who became "clumsy," with a tendency to fall over, 10 days after MMR vaccination. Over the next 2 weeks she became progressively more weak, and was unable to stand without support. Her cough and cry became weak with inability to swallow. She required nasogastric feeding for 4 weeks (Morris & Rylance, 1994).

. **Deafness** caused by nerve damage following MMR vaccine has been reported by many authors. A 7-year-old girl developed total deafness in the left ear 11 days after MMR vaccine. She did not recover (Nabe-Nielsen & Walter, 1988). A 3-year-old girl was diagnosed with moderate to severe bilateral deafness, accompanied by muscle incoordination, attributed to an illness 10 days following MMR vaccination (Brodsky & Stanievich, 1985). A 27-year-old woman developed joint pain, fever, headache, and gait unsteadiness beginning 3 days after measles and rubella vaccination. Progressive hearing loss began 22 days following vaccination. Profound and permanent bilateral hearing loss resulted (Hulbert *et al.*, 1991). A recent review reported six additional cases of profound hearing loss attributed to MMR vaccine in 1 to 6-year-old children (Stewart & Prabhu, 1993).

Optic neuritis accompanied by blindness or partial vision loss has also occurred following MMR vaccination. A 6-year-old boy developed optic neuritis 18 days after MMR injection. He recovered fully after several weeks (Kazarian & Gager, 1978). Marshall and colleagues reported the following case.

> A 16-month-old baby girl ... had been previously healthy and developmentally normal.... In September, 1983, 14 days after measles, mumps, and rubella vaccination, she had subjective fever, cough, conjunctival injection, and a generalized macular erythematous rash. Two days later, the majority of these symptoms abated, but the conjunctival injection worsened, her pupils became dilated, and she began walking into objects.... On admission to the hospital, examination revealed a vigorous toddler who would not reach for objects and had only minimal light perception. Ophthalmologic examination showed a diffuse chorioretinitis with perivascular retinal edema, mild papilledema, and a stellate macular configuration.... Repeat fundoscopic [eye] examination several days later demonstrated evolution into a "salt and pepper" pigmentary pattern distributed radially along the retinal veins. These changes were most consistent with measles retinopathy.... On follow-up examination 7 months later,

her visual acuity had improved; she was able to ambulate freely but still sat close to the television set and held objects close to her face. Fundoscopic examination revealed macular scarring (Marshall *et al.*, 1985).

Thrombocytopenia, a decrease in blood platelets responsible for blood clotting with accompanying spontaneous bleeding, has been acknowledged by the Vaccine Safety Committee as an adverse reaction to measles vaccine, based on overwhelming evidence (Institute of Medicine, 1994). During early research on the measles vaccine, it was discovered that vaccination resulted in a dramatic decrease of platelet counts in 86 percent of vaccinated subjects (Oski & Naiman, 1966).

Many clinical case reports have confirmed the incidence of thrombocytopenia following measles vaccination. Swedish health authorities received reports of 16 cases of thrombocytopenia following MMR vaccination in a three year observation period between 1982 and 1984 (Bottiger *et al.*, 1987). Eleven cases of thrombocytopenia occurred following measles vaccination between 1976 and 1989 in Germany (Fescharek *et al.*, 1990). In Canada, a passive surveillance system received reports of 5 thrombocytopenia cases following MMR vaccination during 1987 (Koch *et al.*, 1989). Finland reported 23 cases of thrombocytopenic purpura occurring within a mean of 19 days of vaccination during a campaign that involved 700,000 children (Nieminen *et al.*, 1993). The VAERS reporting system received 7 case reports of thrombocytopenia following measles or MMR given alone during the period 1990–1992 (Institute of Medicine, 1994).

Anaphylaxis, a severe, acute, systemic, and potentially fatal allergic reaction, has occurred following measles and MMR vaccines. Many reports have documented these reactions. Egg proteins contained in the measles and mumps vaccines may play a role in severe hypersensitivity reactions, since some individuals are exquisitely sensitive to eggs. However, other components of live attenuated virus vaccines, especially the antibiotics contained in these preparations, have been implicated in triggering severe allergic reactions,.

In a report from England, 9 reactions categorized as anaphylaxis with collapse occurred following measles vaccine during a 7 year period (Pollock & Morris, 1983). The Drug Reactions Advisory Committee of Australia received 15 reports of reactions occurring within 30 minutes of measles vaccination during the period 1980–1982

(McEwen, 1983). A measles vaccine grown in monkey kidney cells rather than chicken embryo cells caused 6 severe hypersensitivity reactions in a Norwegian report (Aukrust *et al.*, 1980). The Canadian passive surveillance system reported 30 allergic reactions to MMR during 1987 (Koch *et al.*, 1989). And 9 cases of possible anaphylactic reactions were reported through VAERS during 1990–1992 (Institute of Medicine, 1994).

A disturbing syndrome of **atypical measles** has occurred in children previously vaccinated. This consists of an illness with exaggerated rash, muscle weakness, peripheral edema, and severe abdominal pain with persistent vomiting (Cherry *et al.*, 1972). These reactions, though rare, have also occurred following vaccination (St. Geme, 1976).

Recent research has shown an association between measles vaccine and **inflammatory bowel disease.** In one study individuals who had received measles vaccine in the 1960s were more likely to suffer from chronic intestinal disease including Crohn's disease (characterized by deep ulcers, holes and thickening of the intestinal lining) and ulcerative colitis thirty years later compared to controls (Thompson *et al.*, 1995). This is not surprising since persistent measles virus infection has been located in intestinal tissue affected by chronic inflammation, particularly in Crohn's-disease-affected bowel (Wakefield *et al.*, 1995). These researchers found an incidence rate of 1 case of inflammatory bowel disease for every 140 persons vaccinated for measles, compared to an incidence of 1 in 400 controls (Thompson *et al.*, 1995).

Measles vaccine has been associated with immune system suppression. This mechanism could explain the severe neurologic symptoms and pathology following measles vaccination. Some evidence exists to suggest immune system depression. For example, after measles vaccine, the number of lymphocytes, a type of white blood cell that fights disease, decreases (Nicholson *et al.*, 1992), and certain lymphocyte functions essential to their role in fighting pathogenic organisms are depressed (Hirsch *et al.*, 1981).

Concerns about immune suppression caused by viral vaccines has led Dr. Richard Moskowitz to propose a possible mechanism for long-term sequelae of measles vaccination and other live-virus vaccines. Various viruses, including measles, are capable of stimulating autoimmune responses if they are stored within the body's own cells over long periods of time. Subacute sclerosing panencephalitis represents an instance of measles virus stimulating a severe autoimmune breakdown after a long period of latency following infection. Since the measles virus can be stored within the body's cells and cause such a devastating process years after natural infection, it seems logical that the measles vaccine could stimulate a similar phenomenon. This is the Moskowitz thesis.

> In the case of the attenuated measles virus, it is not difficult to imagine that introducing it directly into the blood would continue to provoke an antibody response for a considerable period of time, which is doubtless the whole point of giving the vaccine; but that eventually, as the virus succeeded in attaining a state of latency within the cell, the antibody response would wane, both because circulating antibodies cannot normally cross the cell membrane, and because they are also powerful immunosuppressive agents in their own right.
>
> The effect of circulating antibody will thereafter be mainly to keep the virus within the cell, i.e., to continue to prevent any acute inflammatory response, until eventually, perhaps under circumstances of accumulated stress or emergency, this precarious balance breaks down, antibodies begin to be produced in large quantities against the cells themselves, and frank auto-immune phenomena of necrosis and tissue destruction supervene (Moskowitz, 1983).

Measles Summary

1. Measles has historically been a common childhood disease with rare complications.
2. Mass vaccination has resulted in a dramatic decline in measles incidence, but outbreaks now occur in older populations and in infants born to women whose immunity from vaccination has deteriorated. Periodic epidemics continue to occur.
3. The vaccine is associated with serious adverse reactions including permanent nervous system damage. Long-term effects are unknown.

Recommendations

Parents must decide whether they are willing to risk the known and unknown adverse effects from the measles vaccine in order to prevent the rare complications of natural measles. I do not recommend the measles vaccine because of the attendant risks, the ability of other healing systems to treat measles infections in children, and the benefits that accrue from lifelong immunity following natural infection.

Mumps

Mumps was a common and very mild disease of childhood that was not even noticed in an estimated 30 percent of cases prior to widespread vaccine use. The illness begins with fever, headache, and fatigue, and within 24 hours the child complains of earache near the lobe of the ear. The next day the salivary gland in front of the ear becomes swollen. Within one to six days, the illness runs its course.

Infection of the testicles, ovaries, and other organs are not unusual, but occur much more commonly in adults. Infection of the testicle occurs in 20 to 30 percent of mumps cases in adolescent or adult males (Philip *et al.*, 1959). Sterility following such an illness is extremely rare. Encephalitis and meningitis complications during epidemic outbreaks occur at a rate of 2 to 4 cases for every 1,000 reported cases of mumps (Centers For Disease Control, 1972). However, only an estimated 70 percent of mumps cases are reported. Deaths from mumps are rare, but much more likely to occur in adults. About half of mumps-associated deaths have been in persons over 20 years old (Centers for Disease Control, 1989g).

Incidence and Vaccine Efficacy

A live mumps virus vaccine was licensed in 1967, and recommended for routine use in 1977. It apparently resulted in a decline in the incidence of mumps cases. Subsequent outbreaks of mumps, however, have caused a re-evaluation of the previous optimistic vaccine success reports. The number of mumps cases had decreased during the early 1980s to 3,000 to 5,000 cases per year, a dramatic decline from the 100,000 cases per year of the early 1970s. However, during 1986, 7,800 cases occurred, and during 1987 there were nearly 13,000 reported mumps cases. During the early 1990s the number of reported cases declined again to around 4,000 cases per year (Centers for Disease Control, 1994).

The most disturbing factor in these statistics is the shift in mumps cases to older age groups who are much more susceptible to the complications of testicular and ovarian infection. During the period 1967–1971, the annual average of cases in persons 15 years of age or older was 8.3 percent; this age group accounted for 38.3 percent of cases in 1987. This represents a greater than eightfold increase (Centers for Disease Control, 1989e). The proportion of mumps in adolescents and adults has remained at that level (34 percent in 1993). Although we are assured that the risk to adolescents is still less than in the pre-vaccine era, this trend is disconcerting. It is thought that the rise in cases among adolescents is due to a lack of vaccination in children born between 1967 and 1977, and not to waning immunity in persons vaccinated previously (Cochi, 1988). Nonetheless, this shift to older populations is worrisome. Mumps in young children is a mild, benign disease. In adolescents and adults, it is a disease associated with more complications. The response of public health authorities is to revaccinate those who are susceptible during adolescent years.

The efficacy of mumps vaccine has ranged from 75 to 95 percent in various studies.

Vaccine Reactions

The mumps vaccine is associated with adverse effects similar to the measles vaccine. Since mumps vaccine is usually administered in combination with measles vaccine, reactions are difficult to accurately attribute to one or the other. Two conditions are associated with the mumps virus and not with measles. These are meningitis and diabetes and other pancreatic diseases. It has been associated with fevers, seizures, encephalitis, and severe, atypical mumps disease.

Meningitis is clearly associated with mumps disease. Cases of aseptic meningitis (not caused by bacteria) reported after administration of mumps vaccine have led researchers around the world to investigate mumps vaccine as a possible cause of meningitis as well. In Canada, the sale of mumps vaccine was suspended in 1990 after the mumps-vaccine virus strain was isolated from 8 children following MMR vaccination (Colville & Pugh, 1992). The rate of virologically confirmed mumps-vaccine associated meningitis was 1 case per 3,800 doses, significantly higher than the incidence of meningitis in children not recently vaccinated. In Yugoslavia, a review of childhood aseptic meningitis cases occurring between 1979 and 1986 revealed that 115 children developed meningitis within 30 days of mumps vaccination. This was an attack rate of 1 case per 1,000 immunized children (Cizman *et al.*, 1989).

In Japan a surveillance program was stimulated during 1989 by public and media attention to mumps-vaccine associated meningitis. This study revealed 311 suspected cases of vaccine associated meningitis. One-third of these suspected cases were later confirmed by laboratory analysis of spinal fluid; however, the authors stated that "Most of the unconfirmed cases were likely to have been vaccine-related, because the two groups (i.e., confirmed and unconfirmed cases) were closely matched in the time of occurrence, the time interval between vaccination and the onset of illness, the age distribution and the clinical manifestation of the illness." Those researchers calculated the incidence rate as 1 in 2,000 people who received MMR (Sugiura & Yamada, 1991). The Vaccine Safety Committee has recognized mumps vaccine as a cause of aseptic meningitis because the vaccine-virus strain can be isolated and positively identified from patients with meningitis following vaccination (Institute of Medicine, 1994).

Diabetes, specifically insulin-dependent diabetes mellitus (IDDM), is characterized by an insufficiency of insulin secretion by the pancreas. Diabetes is thought to arise in response to both genetic and environmental factors. Viruses represent one of the most important environmental triggers of diabetes (Maclaren & Atkinson, 1992). Many studies have proven that natural mumps infection causes pancreatitis (infection of the pancreas) and stimulates the onset of diabetes. This has been shown in the reports of clusters of diabetes following epidemics of mumps disease (Dacou-Voutetakis *et al.*, 1974) and in large epidemiologic studies that demonstrate parallel curves between outbreaks of mumps disease and new cases of diabetes (Sultz *et al.*, 1975).

Mumps vaccination has similarly stimulated the onset of diabetes. The postulated mechanisms of diabetes onset that include autoimmune processes or persistent infection suggest that there may be a prolonged interval between vaccination and the onset of diabetic symptoms (Institute of Medicine, 1994). Nonetheless, many cases of diabetes have been reported following recent mumps vaccination.

One study revealed 20 cases of diabetes occurring after mumps vaccine given during the period 1976 through 1989 in Germany. Twelve cases began within 30 days of vaccination (Fescharek *et al.*, 1990). Another report included 7 children who developed diabetes in the second to fourth week following mumps vaccination (Helmke *et al.*, 1986). A third report cited 3 cases of diabetes beginning 10 days to 3 weeks after mumps vaccination (Otten *et al.*, 1984). Five cases of diabetes following receipt of MMR or mumps vaccine were reported through VAERS during the period 1990–1992 (Institute of Medicine, 1994). During interviews with 112 parents of diabetic children in Erie County, New York, the onset of diabetes was noted by parents to follow mumps disease in almost 50 percent of the children and by mumps vaccination in 11 percent (Sultz *et al.*, 1975).

Several individual cases of diabetes after mumps vaccination have been reported, and one case of pancreatitis occurred in a 19-year-old woman 11 days after MMR vaccination accompanied by abdominal pain and vomiting, and confirmed by abnormal pancreatic enzyme levels on blood tests (Adler *et al.*, 1991). The Vaccine Safety Committee declined to accept diabetes as a consequence of mumps vaccine despite these reports (Institute of Medicine, 1994).

Mumps Summary

1. Mumps is generally a benign disease of children. Complications of mumps do occur, but an estimated 30 percent of cases go unnoticed.
2. Mumps has increasingly become a disease of adolescents and adults since the widespread use of the vaccine.
3. Complications of mumps occur much more frequently in adults.
4. The vaccine has caused significant adverse reactions, including vaccine associated meningitis, in as many as 1 per 1,000 doses.

Recommendations

Use of the mumps vaccine, which has been associated with serious adverse effects, seems unjustifiable. Administering the vaccine during adolescence may simply prolong the problem of waning immunity, and shift the disease and its complications to an even older population.

Rubella (German Measles)

Rubella is a mild childhood illness that consists of fever, rash and tiredness lasting for a few days. It has no serious complications except in very rare instances.

The purpose of vaccination is to prevent pregnant women from contracting rubella, since abortion, stillbirths, and deformities can result from illness during the first three months of pregnancy. Between 20 and 50 percent of babies born to women who contract rubella during pregnancy will have birth defects (eye defects, deafness, mental retardation). This vaccine is unique in that children are vaccinated to interrupt circulation of the virus and reduce the risk of exposure to susceptible pregnant women.

Prevention of rubella using the live-virus vaccine can be accomplished in one of two ways: 1. vaccinate susceptible women of childbearing age, or 2. vaccinate preschool and school-age children to prevent disease transmission. The question has persistently arisen whether the rubella vaccine should be given to children or to susceptible adolescent and adult women, with many experts on both sides of this controversy.

Drs. Otto Sieber and Vincent Fulginiti, recognized vaccine experts, argued against routine vaccination of children (Fulginiti, 1976; Sieber & Fulginiti, 1977). When reports appeared that antibody titers decreased after childhood rubella vaccination, they stated, "one might argue that immunization of adolescents or adults might be a more appropriate strategy than our current emphasis upon vaccination of infants...." If the protective effect of the vaccine decreases over time, then a girl who is vaccinated during childhood may become susceptible once again as an adult. If the vaccine has significant adverse effects, then vaccinated children could be needlessly exposed to this risk. Both of these factors argue against the use of rubella vaccine in children.

Another reason for vaccination of susceptible adult women rather than children was put forward by Dr. Stephen Schoenbaum and colleagues in 1975, in the *Journal of the American Medical Association*. They discovered that children may not be the major source of rubella spread to pregnant women. They tested a hypothesis:

> If children were an important source of contagion for pregnant women, it should be reflected by one of the following: First, the percentage of women with detectable antibody titers, signifying previous experience with rubella, should rise with increasing parity [number of children born to a woman] more than one would expect on the basis of age alone. Second, the incidence of rubella among susceptible pregnant women should increase with increasing parity and should be reflected by an increasing frequency of babies with rubella syndrome among children born of later pregnancies.

In other words, mothers should show evidence of more exposure to rubella than other women. Their study found the opposite to be true.

> To summarize the serologic data, there was no evidence of a decrease in susceptibility with increasing parity. These data, therefore, offer no support for the presumption that the number of susceptible adult women materially decreases after the first pregnancy.... This finding is consistent with the concept that most persons who contract rubella as adults do so through contact with other adults (Schoenbaum *et al.*, 1975).

If children are not the primary source of infection for pregnant women, then children should not be targeted for prevention. They come to the logical conclusion that "We ... would prefer the alternative policy of selectively and efficiently vaccinating adolescent girls."

Incidence

The incidence of rubella and congenital rubella syndrome (infants with defects due to maternal infections) has declined dramatically since the vaccine was licensed in 1969. Previous levels of 20,000 to 60,000 reported cases of rubella per year declined to several hundred per year in the 1980s. During 1988, 221 cases of rubella were reported. In 1987, 3 indigenous cases of congenital rubella syndrome were reported, and only 1 was reported in 1988 (Centers for Disease Control, 1989f).

Vaccine efficacy

The protective effect of rubella vaccine has been estimated as 77 percent in one study (Hough *et al.*, 1979). A continuing concern is the gradual reduction in an individual's antibody titer following rubella vaccination. The effectiveness of the vaccine may decrease, so that women who were not susceptible as children become susceptible again as adults. In fact, the disease has shifted to older age groups. During the three-year period before vaccine licensure (1966–1968), 23 percent of rubella cases occurred among persons 15 years of age or older. In 1987, 48 percent of cases occurred in persons 15 or more years old (Centers for Disease Control, 1989f). Serologic surveys of postpubertal populations have found that rates of rubella susceptibility are comparable to the prevaccine years (10 to 20 percent lack evidence of immunity) (Crowder *et al.*, 1987; Bart *et al.*, 1985). The proposed solution to this problem of shifting age-occurrence has again been to revaccinate susceptible women of childbearing age.

Vaccine reactions

Adverse effects of the rubella vaccine include encephalitis-type symptoms, meningitis, and Guillain-Barré syndrome (muscle paralysis and sensory nerve deficits). In addition, at least 12 to 20 percent of women develop arthritis symptoms after receiving the vaccine. These may begin several weeks after the administration of vaccine (Fulginiti, 1976). They may persist for weeks, months, or years. In some cases, women develop rheumatoid arthritis, which continues throughout their lives.

Many studies since the 1960s have proven that rubella vaccine causes **acute arthritis** in both children and adults. Joint pain and arthritis occur in 10 to 40 percent of women after vaccination, and less often in children. One study showed that 25 percent of women in their 20s and 50 percent of those aged 25 to 33 had joint symptoms following rubella vaccination (Swartz et al., 1971). In another study, acute arthritis occurred in 46 percent of women above age 25 years (Weibel et al., 1972). No children involved in these 2 small studies developed arthritis.

Chronic persistent arthritis occurs following both natural rubella infection and rubella vaccination. Natural rubella has been associated with chronic arthritis, as evidenced in several studies. For example, rubella virus antigen was demonstrated in joint cavities of one-third of patients with juvenile rheumatoid arthritis (Ogra et al., 1975), and the virus was isolated from blood cells or joint fluid in one-third of children with chronic rheumatic disease (Chantler et al., 1985). Many cases of recurrent or persistent arthritis have been reported in the medical literature following rubella vaccination. One study reported 11 children with recurrent arthritis 36 months after vaccination (Thompson et al., 1973). Arthritis persisting for at least 2 to 7 years has been reported in several women following rubella vaccine injection (Tingle et al., 1984; Tingle et al., 1985). The author has seen a case of rheumatoid arthritis with joint destruction that began after rubella vaccination and has persisted for over 20 years.

One study compared the effects of natural rubella infection in 46 people with the effects of rubella vaccination in a second group of 44 women. In the group with natural rubella, 65 percent had acute arthritis or joint pain. Eighteen months later, 30 percent of the women and 8 percent of the men had joint symptoms. In the vaccinated group, 55 percent had arthritis or joint pain within 4 weeks, and 5 percent had persistent joint symptoms 18 months later (Tingle et al., 1986). In their analysis of these and other studies, the Vaccine Safety Committee concluded that rubella vaccine causes acute and chronic arthritis (Institute of Medicine, 1991).

Various types of **central and peripheral nervous system disorders** have been frequently reported to follow rubella vaccination. One study examined 299 reported cases of peripheral neuropathies, including 10 children with symptoms that persisted for more than 32 months. That study found an incidence of 2.2 cases of neuropathies per 1,000 doses of one vaccine virus strain, and 0.1 per 1,000 doses of a second strain (Schaffner *et al.,* 1974). Other individual cases have been scattered through the literature. These include reports of cases of nerve pain and numbness, carpal tunnel syndrome, 2 cases of Guillain-Barré syndrome, and 3 cases of transverse myelitis (Institute of Medicine, 1991).

The following case was reported in the *American Journal of Diseases of Children.*

> A 20-month-old white boy was well until ten days after inoculation with the combined mumps-rubella vaccine. Initial complaints were the inability to stand on the left leg and pain in all extremities. The weakness progressed to include both legs and ascended to involve all extremities.... Examination revealed an apprehensive child with a complete flaccid paralysis of all extremities and inability to hold his head up. The patient had marked soft tissue tenderness of all extremities. Neurologic evaluation revealed no muscle stretch reflexes.... Over a three-month period he completely recovered all motor functions (Gunderman, 1973).

This case is similar to other descriptions of weakness or paralysis of extremities, loss of sensation, and difficulty walking in other children who reacted to the rubella vaccine (Kilroy, 1970; Gilmartin *et al.,* 1972).

A 13-year-old boy developed **Guillain-Barré syndrome** 3 weeks after he received MMR and booster doses of diphtheria, tetanus, and oral polio vaccines. Symptoms began with tingling in the feet and muscular weakness, which progressed for 2 weeks, when he could still walk but could not stand up or climb stairs without assistance. He recovered after a month. Blood tests revealed high levels of rubella antibody consistent with rubella infection. No other symptoms of rubella occurred, and his illness was attributed to the rubella vaccination (Mühlebach-Sponer *et al.,* 1994).

Several case reports have indicated an association between rubella and **thrombocytopenia,** decrease of blood platelets with consequent spontaneous bleeding. Four cases were reported within 10 days to 3 weeks of rubella vaccination. A 26-year-old woman developed thrombocytopenia with bleeding into the skin and mucus membranes, and marked reduction in blood platelets after rubella vaccination (Bartos, 1972). Other cases involved the MMR vaccine, and reactions were impossible to distinguish between measles and rubella.

Rubella Summary

1. Rubella is a mild childhood disease which requires no treatment.
2. A woman who contracts rubella during the first three months of pregnancy risks abortion, miscarriage, or birth defects in her child.
3. Rubella incidence has shifted to older age groups since widespread vaccination.
4. Rubella vaccine is associated with significant adverse effects, including arthritis and central nervous system disorders.

Recommendations

Parents have three options: avoid the vaccine entirely; vaccinate their child against rubella; or test girls for antibodies at adolescence or before considering pregnancy, and decide whether to vaccinate then. Since a child's health is not compromised by contracting rubella, there is no advantage to the child from vaccination.

Every adolescent girl and woman of childbearing age should have a blood test for immunity to rubella. If they do not have evidence of immunity, then they should decide whether they wish to have the vaccine. Susceptible women who decline the vaccine should attempt to avoid exposure to children with colds, fevers, and rashes during the first three months of pregnancy. Again, the consideration is whether the possible adverse effects of the vaccine are worth prevention of problems during pregnancy. Avoidance of the vaccine during childhood will eliminate the risk of untoward vaccine reactions in your child.

Haemophilus Influenzae
Type B (Hib) Meningitis

Haemophilus influenzae bacterial infections occur frequently in childhood, accounting for a large percentage of common sinus, throat, and ear infections. They usually resolve on their own without treatment. However, one strain of *Haemophilus,* the type b encapsulated strain, is capable of causing invasion of infections to deeper levels in the body, particularly the spinal fluid, lungs, heart, and blood. Vaccines have been developed because *Haemophilus* can cause meningitis, pneumonia, epiglottitis, and other complications. The bacteria has no relationship to influenza. It was named *influenzae* because early researchers found the bacteria in people with flu, but did not recognize until later that *Haemophilus* is a normal resident of mucus membranes.

Meningitis in children often begins with flu-like symptoms including fever, headache, nausea and vomiting, tiredness, and irritability. This may be followed by a change in alertness, stiff neck, and seizures. Between 20 and 30 percent of children with bacterial meningitis have seizures. Arthritis, pericarditis, and pneumonia are common complications (Kaplan & Fishman, 1988). Disease of sudden onset with rapid progression is usually associated with a different bacteria, *Neisseria meningitidis,* which has a much higher risk of death. A sudden change in level of alertness or severe headache in children is cause for concern.

Mortality from Hib meningitis is 3 to 8 percent (Sell, 1987). Sensorineural (permanent) hearing loss occurs in approximately 10 percent of meningitis cases (Dodge *et al.*, 1984), though this is most common with pneumococcal meningitis. Appropriate treatment of Hib meningitis includes the use of a cephalosporin (or other) antibiotic, administered intravenously. Some organisms have proven resistant to various antibiotics.

Several studies have observed long-term cognitive effects of previous *Haemophilus influenzae* meningitis on children. Most recent studies have found no differences in IQ scores or academic success of children with a history of meningitis compared to their sibling controls (Tejani *et al.*, 1982; Feldman & Michaels, 1988; R.D. Feigin & P.R. Dodge, unpublished data). But several previously conducted studies did find that learning disabilities, reading problems, and lower IQ scores occurred more frequently in postmeningitic children compared to randomly selected peer-group controls (Sell *et al.*, 1972; Pate, 1972). This may indicate that Hib meningitis is associated with learning problems, but the validity of this association is still in question.

Incidence

The estimated incidence of Hib meningitis is 8,000 to 15,000 cases per year. Native American and Eskimo children are particularly susceptible to Hib meningitis. Incidence has increased over the past three decades. Some observers associate this increase with the administration of other vaccines and their apparent ability to impair immune system resistance. Although this link has not been proven, the tendency of vaccines to cause neurologic complications has raised suspicions that central nervous system infections occur more frequently as a direct result of DTP and measles vaccine (Coulter, 1990).

Approximately 1 in 350 children younger than 5 years of age develops Hib meningitis (Sell, 1987). Children under 6 months are protected by maternal antibodies, and breastfeeding reduces incidence rates (Istre *et al.*, 1985; Cochi *et al.*, 1986). The peak incidence of meningitis occurs in children 6 to 7 months of age. The attack rate decreases rapidly with increasing age. Fifty percent of cases occur in infants under 1 year of age. Only 25 to 30 percent of cases occur in children over 18 months old (Broome, 1987).

The congregation of infants in day care settings creates a significantly higher risk of infection (Istre *et al.*, 1985; Cochi *et al.*, 1986; Fleming *et al.*, 1985). In one study, 50 percent of all invasive disease caused by *H. influenzae* type b was attributable to day care settings (Cochi *et al.*, 1986). In these studies more of the children with Hib had attended day care than children without the disease. Later studies attempting to show the transmission of Hib in day care settings did not reveal a pattern of disease spread between children. Two studies failed to find cases of *H. influenzae* invasive disease in contacts of children with primary infections in day care settings (Osterholm *et al.*, 1987; Murphy *et al.*, 1987).

Vaccine efficacy

Several different *Haemophilus influenzae* type b (Hib) vaccines are manufactured. Efficacy studies for the newer vaccines have only been published since 1987, and conclusions about the comparative effectiveness of the vaccines based on these studies are tentative. The quality of studies varies, and the findings can only be applied to the specific form of the vaccine being evaluated.

In 1985 the first Hib vaccine, a purified form of the polysaccharide capsule (called PRP, from the chemical name of the capsular substance), was licensed. The PRP vaccine was not effective in children under 24 months old, and these children represented 80 percent of Hib meningitis cases (Ward, 1987). The development of the vaccine was enthusiastically heralded as a great step in prevention of Hib invasive disease, but hopes for its success were soon dashed.

The effectiveness of the PRP vaccine was called into question by a case-control study published in the *Journal of the American Medical Association.* This study found that 41 percent of Hib cases occurred in vaccinated children. The vaccine's protective efficacy was minus 58 percent. In other words, children were much more likely to get the disease if they had received the vaccine (Osterholm *et al.*, 1988). Apparently the vaccine had lowered their resistance and created an environment that encouraged the spread of the disease to the nervous system. This is precisely what one would predict if the vaccines do suppress immune system function.

In other studies, vaccine efficacy ranged from 41 to 88 percent.

An active surveillance study which included a population of 2.5 million children under five years of age identified 1,444 cases of invasive Hib disease. Vaccine efficacy in this group was found to be 62 percent compared to controls—again a much lower figure than expected by researchers (Harrison *et al.*, 1989). As improved forms of vaccine were developed, the PRP vaccine was abandoned.

Vaccine researchers found that when the PRP form of the vaccine was joined to a protein carrier, then the vaccine was more effective, and developed antibody responses in younger children. These "conjugated" forms are now used beginning in infancy. In 1990, the first conjugate vaccines were licensed for use beginning at 2 months of age.

Evaluating the efficacy of the conjugate vaccines has been complicated by the different versions of protein carriers studied in varied populations with several different types of study methods. The technology of conjugate vaccines has developed rapidly over a short period of time. Several conjugate vaccines have been rushed through licensure, some with only one or two efficacy trials. The field trials evaluating the PRP-T conjugate vaccine in 5,200 infants were terminated early because another Hib vaccine was licensed during the study period, and all controls subsequently received the new Hib vaccine (Vadheim *et al.*, 1993). PRP-T was licensed nonetheless, despite the findings in this study that PRP-T vaccine caused a higher incidence of seizures, crying, and high fevers than the control vaccines in these children (Vadheim *et al.*, 1993).

The dismal failure of the previous unconjugated PRP vaccine spurred the adoption of the newer conjugate versions, sometimes with only one or two efficacy trials. The effectiveness of the various conjugate vaccines as measured in these studies has varied. For example, the PRP-D conjugate vaccine showed an efficacy of 74 to 96 percent in various studies (Centers for Disease Control, 1993), but in a study of Alaskan Natives the efficacy was only 35 percent, indicating that it did not confer immunity. The vaccine proved entirely ineffective in either stimulating protective antibody levels or preventing Hib disease in these infants (Ward *et al.*, 1990). The authors eliminated the possibility that genetic factors played a role in this vaccine failure because they detected no differences in genetic markers that could distinguish susceptibility to Hib disease in Alaskan

Natives compared to controls (Petersen *et al.,* 1987). They concluded, "the findings of this study indicate that three doses of PRP-D vaccine induce marginal immune responses in young infants, and in infants at high risk three doses fail to provide significant protection. The most likely reason for these results is an intrinsic limitation in the immunogenicity of the PRP-D vaccine, at least in young infants" (Ward *et al.,* 1990).

In another study, 90 percent of children vaccinated with the PRP-D conjugate vaccine responded with antibody levels considered to be protective, but only 60 percent produced levels of antibody indicating long-term protection (Berkowitz *et al.,* 1987). Nonetheless, millions of children are vaccinated with PRP-D. Other conjugate vaccines (PRP-OMP and HbOC) have shown high levels of efficacy in the few trials conducted. One study of the PRP-OMP conjugate vaccine showed a 93 percent efficacy (Santosham *et al.,* 1991). The HbOC vaccine was evaluated in two studies that showed a 100 percent (Black *et al.,* 1990) and 97 percent (Eskola *et al.,* 1990) level of efficacy. It must be remembered, however, that these studies were each conducted over a one- or two-year period. The continuing protective effect of Hib vaccines is unknown because of their short history.

Regardless of the reported efficacy rates of conjugate vaccines, they have quickly been credited with a drop in reported cases of Hib-invasive disease. One report claimed that "Hib disease has been nearly eradicated in a fully immunized population" (children enrolled in a particular HMO health plan). These authors report that the incidence of Hib disease for infants decreased in Los Angeles the year *prior* to the licensure of vaccine for this age group, yet they audaciously attribute this declining incidence of Hib during that year (1990) to the vaccine. They speculated that this decline could be due to less transmission of Hib from older children who *were* vaccinated.

After licensure of Hib vaccine for infants in 1990, the incidence of Hib disease in Los Angeles infants continued to decline in the study period (1991 and 1992) although the rate of fully vaccinated infants was only 14 percent of 6- to 17-month-old children and 40 percent of 1- to 5-month-old children in 1991, increasing to less than 60 percent in 1992 (Vadheim *et al.,* 1994).

The argument that declining disease incidence is caused by the introduction of vaccine in a community may or may not be true.

Many epidemiological factors could contribute to the decline of a highly infectious disease. The triumphant title of that article, "Eradication of Hib Disease," has proven to be premature in reference to other diseases whose incidence also waxes and wanes during vaccination campaign years.

Similar spectacular results of the Hib vaccine campaign have been claimed in Finland, where over 90 percent of infants are vaccinated. During the 1950s, the incidence of Hib meningitis in greater Helsinki averaged 8 cases per year. This increased to an average of 22 cases per year during the period 1976–1985. After the introduction of Hib vaccine in 1985, the incidence declined to the previous levels of 3 to 9 cases per year (Peltola *et al.*, 1992). Comparable declines in Hib disease were reported In Minnesota (85 percent decline) and Dallas, Texas (92 percent decline); however, the decline in Dallas Hib cases began prior to the introduction of vaccination, and efficacy studies in Minnesota showed Hib vaccines to be ineffective (Murphy *et al.*, 1993).These figures may merely indicate a peak of Hib meningitis cases in the 1980s that began to decline prior to and coincident with the introduction of Hib vaccination. The celebration of Hib vaccine effectiveness may need to wait for more definitive and long-term studies.

Vaccine reactions

Evaluating reactions to the Hib conjugate vaccines presents problems because Hib vaccines are given together with the DTP vaccines, sometimes in the same shot. Reactions, therefore, could be attributable to any of these four vaccines. The most reliable indications that Hib vaccines cause significant reactions come from field trials where the vaccine is given alone. The withdrawn PRP vaccine caused significant adverse effects including seizures, anaphylactoid allergic reactions, serum sickness-like reactions (joint pain, rashes, and edema), and one death within 4 hours of vaccination. These effects were reviewed in a study of 152 spontaneous reports of vaccine reactions submitted to the FDA during the first year of vaccine availability, 1985–1986 (Milstien *et al.*, 1987). Only reactions to the newer conjugate vaccine are reviewed here.

The most common and potentially significant Hib vaccine reaction has been the **increased incidence of Hib disease** following vaccination. The older PRP vaccine caused Hib disease within the first 7 days following vaccination in children over 18 months of age. This was confirmed in 4 case-control studies conducted in 1988 that all found a 2- to 6-times increased chance of contracting Hib disease in the first week after vaccination compared to controls (Black *et al.*, 1988; Harrison *et al.*, 1988; Osterholm *et al.*, 1988; Shapiro *et al.*, 1988).

The new conjugate vaccines also cause a decline in antibody levels immediately following vaccination (Daum *et al.*, 1989). Ten cases of early Hib disease following vaccination with conjugate vaccines were reported through VAERS between 1990 and 1992. All cases occurred within 5 days of vaccination. Investigators have postulated that increased susceptibility to infection in the immediate post-vaccination period might be related either to a transient decrease in pre-existing antibody or to transient suppression of antibody synthesis (Marchant *et al.*, 1989; Sood & Daum, 1990).

The conjugate vaccines have been associated with the onset of **Guillain-Barré syndrome (GBS).** Many cases have been reported in the medical literature and through VAERS. Some of these children received other vaccines concurrently, but several cases occurred when the Hib vaccine was given alone. A 4-year-old girl developed progressive weakness of the legs, pain in the legs and feet and gradual inability to walk 10 days after Hib vaccination. On the fifth day she had swallowing difficulties, facial weakness, and a monotonous voice. Her symptoms gradually improved, and within 3 weeks she could walk with help (Gervaix *et al.*, 1993). Two cases were reported after PRP-D alone (D'Cruz, 1989), and three cases following the HbOC conjugate vaccine were reported through VAERS prior to 1992 (Institute of Medicine, 1994).

Cases of **transverse myelitis,** a paralyzing disease of the spinal cord, following Hib vaccine have been reported through VAERS. One child developed a 105° temperature, extreme floppiness, and toxic appearance within 24 hours of the HbOC conjugate vaccine given alone. Two other children received HbOC accompanied by DTP and OPV vaccination. One of these children developed persistent paralysis and spinal cord lesions. The other baby was unable to crawl following vaccination. Further details were not presented (Institute of Medicine, 1994).

In a study examining the safety of Hib conjugate vaccine (PRP-T) compared to hepatitis B vaccine, in which all infants were also given DTP, five infants developed **seizures** within 48 hours of vaccination in the PRP-T group, compared to none in the control group (Vadheim *et al.*, 1993). Three additional infants had seizures between 3 and 14 days after Hib vaccination, compared to 2 infants who received hepatitis B. Two children in the PRP-T group died from possible vaccine reactions. One child developed symptoms of muscle weakness 1 week after vaccination, which progressed to muscle wasting over the next 5 months and eventually resulted in death at 7 months of age. A second child died at 14 months from central nervous system demyelination, a frequently encountered reaction to vaccines. Since these children all received DTP and OPV concurrently with the Hib vaccine, it is difficult to attribute their reactions to Hib vaccination alone. However, the significant differences in the two groups suggests that the Hib vaccine could have caused these reactions, or potentiated the adverse reaction to DTP.

Thrombocytopenia, a decrease in blood platelets responsible for clotting and consequent spontaneous bleeding, has been reported following Hib conjugate vaccination. Five cases of thrombocytopenia were reported in VAERS between 1990 and 1992 in children who also received DTP or MMR in addition to Hib vaccines (Institute of Medicine, 1994). In an early research study of 15 subjects who received the PRP-D conjugate vaccine, extensive blood testing of vaccine recipients revealed an asymptomatic fall in blood platelet count in one study subject (Granoff *et al.*, 1984). A postmarketing survey of the earlier PRP vaccine revealed 3 cases of low platelet counts or bleeding into the skin following Hib vaccination (Milstien *et al.*, 1987).

Haemophilus influenzae *b (Hib)* *Meningitis Summary*

1. Hib meningitis is a potentially life-threatening disease, and long-term sequelae of infections (hearing loss, learning disabilities) do occur.
2. Long-term effectiveness of the vaccines has not been determined, and reports of short-term effectiveness vary considerably.
3. Serious vaccine-associated reactions have been reported.
4. The vaccine has been associated with an increased susceptibility to Hib meningitis in the first week following vaccination.

Recommendations

Ironically, this new vaccine, relatively untested and questionably effective, presents the most difficult decision for parents. Meningitis is not a mild childhood disease. *Haemophilus* meningitis is not uncommon. Parents must make a choice about the Hib vaccine based on a few facts and vague uncertainties about the vaccine.

One issue remains clear: if a child stays home with a parent in the first 12 to 18 months of life, when Hib disease occurs most often, then the likelihood of exposure decreases dramatically compared to a child who attends a large day care center.

Parents should weigh the likelihood of exposure against their feelings about the known adverse effects of Hib vaccine, including the ability of the vaccine to suppress immune system function and cause an increased susceptibility to Hib disease. A parent's philosophy about immune system competence, unknown effects of vaccines, and the politics of vaccine campaign promotion will always enter into the decision process when a new vaccine is marketed for a serious disease. New vaccines are always experiments. The inflated claims and hyperbolic enthusiasm that accompany a marketing campaign should not lull parents into consenting to a risky experiment on their child.

Hepatitis B

Hepatitis is a viral infection usually acquired during adolescence or adulthood as a result of sexual contact, injection drug use, or occupational or household exposure. Infants born to hepatitis B infected mothers are at high risk of contracting hepatitis. The risk of an infant acquiring hepatitis depends on the mother's hepatitis B antigen status. Infants who become infected at birth have a 90 percent risk of chronic infection, and up to 25 percent will die of chronic liver disease as adults (Beasley & Hwang, 1984). Children do not commonly contract hepatitis except through family exposure.

Hepatitis B infection usually goes unnoticed. Acute infection may have no symptoms, or it may be characterized by flu-like symptoms—weakness, loss of appetite, diarrhea and right upper abdomen pain. Jaundice may accompany these symptoms, with dark urine, light-colored stools, and yellowing of the eyes and skin. Most cases recover fully. In 5 to 10 percent of cases, infection can persist for many years in a chronic form and cause liver damage or liver cancer. In rare cases of acute infections, liver failure may occur with possible coma and death. Approximately 1 to 3 percent of identified hepatitis B cases progress to liver failure.

Screening pregnant women for HBsAg (hepatitis B surface antigen) will identify those infants at risk of acquiring hepatitis. If a mother is HBsAg negative, then it is extremely unlikely that a child will contract hepatitis B.

171

Incidence

The Centers for Disease Control estimate that there are 200,000 to 300,000 new cases of hepatitis B yearly in the United States. However this figure has been disputed. The CDC has maintained the quarter of a million figure since 1985, but reported cases had dropped by 38 percent as of 1992. No actual "empirical" figures were supplied by the CDC to justify their "extrapolated" estimate (Experts question, 1990). A corrected estimation of 33,000 to 165,000 annual cases has been proposed (McEwen, 1993). Fewer than 1 percent of hepatitis B cases occur in children younger than 15 years (Alter *et al.*, 1990).

Vaccine strategy

Hepatitis B vaccine (HBV) has only recently been recommended for children. Prior to the 1991 CDC recommendation for universal vaccination of children beginning at birth, medical providers used the vaccine primarily for the following high-risk groups: people with multiple sex partners, health care workers, populations with a high incidence of hepatitis, users of illicit injectable drugs, etc. This strategy did not lower the incidence of hepatitis B. The failure of the hepatitis vaccine strategy was attributed to the difficulty getting high-risk populations to comply (Centers for Disease Control, 1991c).

Not everyone agreed with the idea of preventing hepatitis in teenagers and adults by vaccinating all infants at birth. Parents often saw no reason to vaccinate their child if they knew the mother was not infected with hepatitis. Why not just give the vaccine to infants whose mothers showed a positive blood test for hepatitis antigen? Since hepatitis is not a childhood disease, the expense and the addition of yet another series of shots to the schedule of 13 to 15 vaccines made little sense. Many physicians agreed. Following the CDC recommendation in 1991 that all infants receive hepatitis vaccine, only 32 percent of pediatricians in North Carolina responding to a survey questionnaire thought the vaccine was warranted for all newborns (Freed *et al.*, 1993). A study to determine whether family practitioners agreed with the new recommendation found similar results (Freed *et al.*, 1993a).

The new policy came under fire for a variety of reasons. The expense of such a project seemed less than cost effective. Family physicians argued, "Given that 4 million infants are born in this country each year, a universal vaccination program costing only $50 per infant will cost $200 million each year. Since the majority of the program's effect will not be seen for 15 to 20 years, the nation will spend $3 to $4 billion before a significant effect on hepatitis B is seen" (Ganiats *et al.*, 1993). Targeting high risk infants and teenagers, it is argued, would provide more immediate and cost effective protection.

Several authors have pointed out the absurdity of vaccinating infants to protect them from a disease of adulthood, since the protective effect of the vaccine decreases significantly over time. When addressing the question of persistent immunity after hepatitis B vaccination, the American Academy of Pediatrics Committee on Infectious Disease members casually remarked that "immunologic memory... persists for at least 10 years in normal adults and infants" (Hall & Halsey, 1992). Yet several studies report consistent declines in hepatitis B antibody. One study found that only 52 percent of vaccinees maintained antibody levels above the recommended level after 4 years (Pasko & Beam, 1990). Another study produced similar findings showing that over 60 percent of vaccine recipients had subprotective levels 4.5 years after vaccination (Street *et al.*, 1990). The CDC recommendations statement admits that "follow-up studies of children vaccinated at birth to prevent perinatal HBV infection have shown that a continued high level of protection from chronic HBV infections persists at least 5 years" (Centers for Disease Control, 1991c).

If protection from the vaccine only lasts 5 years, and hepatitis is a disease of adults, what is the point of vaccinating children? I would propose that the point is selling more vaccine. Vaccinated infants obviously will need a booster at adolescence. How much more vaccine will be sold if everyone were vaccinated twice in their lives? The CDC statement affirms that booster doses of vaccine are not recommended, but then admits, "the possible need for booster doses will be assessed as additional information becomes available." Many authors ask, "Why not just vaccinate the adolescents?"

Vaccine policy officials had given up on vaccinating adolescents. The American Academy of Pediatrics Committee on Infectious Disease decided to vaccinate infants because "achieving adequate coverage and compliance [in adolescents] was thought to be problematic" (Hall & Halsey, 1992). The logic in this argument has been questioned by other physicians: "What about the CDC's argument that teenagers are too hard to vaccinate? Would you really implement a childhood vaccination program that may not work when needed just because the program is convenient?" (Ganiats *et al.,* 1993). If you can't get adolescents to take the primary series, what makes anyone think they will accept a booster?

Nonetheless, the program to vaccinate all children beginning at birth continues. The vaccine campaign of infants began in 1991. Each child now receives three doses of vaccine. In 2020 these children will be adults. Then we may have some follow-up to see if the strategy worked. In the meantime, the cost of giving these vaccines remains enormous in terms of financial commitment and adverse effects.

Vaccine efficacy

How effective is the hepatitis B vaccine? Two different types of vaccines have been developed. A plasma-derived vaccine was licensed by the FDA in 1981 and subsequently abandoned because of fears that vaccine obtained from human serum could transmit unrecognized viruses, particularly HIV (Institute of Medicine, 1994). The first synthetic recombinant vaccines were licensed in 1986. Only the plasma cell vaccines have been evaluated for duration of vaccine effectiveness. Those studies have proven that the vaccine is 80 to 95 percent effective in preventing HBV infection and clinical hepatitis.

Different individuals mount different levels of antibody response to the vaccine, and then these antibody levels steadily decline. It is generally assumed, based on study results, that immunity persists for 5 to 9 years following the three-dose series of vaccine (Stevens *et al.,* 1992). Some of these studies may be methodologically flawed because of inadequate follow-up, but it is clear that the vaccine does protect individuals at risk, including children born to hepatitis antigen-positive mothers (Lo *et al.,* 1988) and homosexual men (Hadler *et al.,* 1986), at least on a short-term basis.

It is not surprising to find reports of vaccine failure sprinkled throughout the medical literature. For example, a 26-year-old man suffered acute hepatitis B infection 2 years after full HBV vaccination (Ballinger & Clark, 1994). A 60-year-old woman on hemodialysis received a kidney transplant 18 months after vaccination with HBV. Six months later she developed hepatitis B. Similarly, a 37-year-old woman contracted hepatitis B five months after receiving a kidney transplant, despite vaccination with HBV one year prior (Goffin *et al.*, 1995).

Hepatitis vaccine has only been available for a relatively short period of time. It is probable that declining levels of antibody in vaccine recipients and continued reports of vaccine failure will result in future recommendations for repeated booster doses with unknown effectiveness, even though experts now decline to recommend booster vaccinations (Hall, 1993).

Vaccine reactions

The CDC assures us that "Hepatitis B vaccines have been shown to be safe when administered to both adults and children" (Centers for Disease Control, 1991c). They mention no adverse reactions among the 8 million people vaccinated prior to 1991. This blatant avoidance of the facts is astounding. Studies and case reports have consistently identified Guillain-Barré syndrome, arthritis, demyelinating nervous system disease, and anaphylaxis as reactions to hepatitis B vaccines. Other types of reactions have been reported as well.

A disturbing number of reported **autoimmune reactions** have occurred following vaccination with HBV. A 39-year-old woman developed jaundice, loss of appetite, tiredness and vomiting 4 weeks after receiving her first dose of recombinant HBV. Antibodies to DNA were detected on blood testing. She recovered within 4 months (Lilic & Ghosh, 1994). Two cases of **thrombocytopenic purpura**, another suspected autoimmune phenomenon that causes bleeding into the skin, mucus membranes, and other organs due to decreased blood platelets required for clotting were reported in the same issue of *Lancet*. A 15-year-old girl developed isolated purpura 4 weeks after receiving the third dose of HBV. A 21-year-old woman developed purpura and an enlarged spleen 3 weeks after receiving the second dose of HBV (Poullin & Gabriel, 1994). A 33-year-old man developed acute abdominal pain, multiple inflamed joints in his hands and feet, chills, and fever two days after HBV vaccination. Blood tests showed decreased platelets and anemia caused by an autoimmune mechanism (Martinez & Domingo, 1992). This combination of hemolytic anemia and thrombocytopenia in the same patient is extremely unusual.

Cases of **Guillain-Barré syndrome (GBS)**, another autoimmune phenomenon, following HBV were identified in a large surveillance study of 850,000 vaccine recipients during the 3 year period 1982 to 1985. This study identified 9 cases of GBS that occurred within 7 weeks of a hepatitis B vaccine dose (Shaw *et al.*, 1988). The rate of GBS incidence in the vaccine group proved to be significantly higher than the background incidence in the general population. Several isolated cases of GBS following hepatitis vaccine have been reported in the medical literature (Ribera & Dutka, 1983; Morris & Butler, 1992). Fourteen cases of GBS were reported to the Vaccine Adverse Event Reporting System (VAERS) during 1990 to 1992 (Institute of Medicine, 1994). Despite these studies and reported cases, the Vaccine Safety Committee declined to recognize a causal relationship between hepatitis B vaccine and GBS (Institute of Medicine, 1994).

Many cases of other **central nervous system demyelinating diseases** following HBV have been reported as well. A 28-year-old woman developed muscular weakness and partial paralysis 6 weeks after receiving HBV. A diagnostic MRI revealed hyperintense lesions in the white matter of the left cerebral hemisphere, indicating multiple sclerosis. A follow-up MRI revealed extension of this lesion, and an additional area of demyelination. At 3 months she remained partially paralyzed (Herroelen *et al.*, 1992). A 26-year-old woman with a previous history of relapsing multiple sclerosis and complete recovery after these episodes received the HBV vaccine. Six weeks later she had a recurrence of multiple sclerosis symptoms, but this time the symptoms did not improve. Four years later she continued to suffer from partial paralysis (Herroelen *et al.*, 1992). An 11-year-old girl developed headache, back pain, leg weakness, and urine retention 3 weeks after a hepatitis vaccine injection. Her muscle weakness of the legs improved, but she was left with apparently permanent inability to normally empty her bladder (Trevisani *et al.*, 1993). Two cases of multiple sclerosis were reported to the Institute of Medicine in 32-year-old and 37-year-old women who developed symptoms 3 and 2 weeks following HBV (Waisbren, 1992). Fourteen additional cases of demyelinating disease were reported in VAERS (Institute of Medicine, 1994). Needless to say, the Vaccine Safety Committee refused to recognize a causal relationship between HBV and any demyelinating disease.

Arthritis following hepatitis vaccine is another well-recognized phenomenon. The Vaccine Adverse Event Reporting System (VAERS) had received 57 well-documented reports of arthritis developing within 2 months after receipt of HBV between 1990 and 1992 (Institute of Medicine, 1994). Other reports have occurred in the literature as well. A 15-year-old girl developed severe pain, swelling, and redness in her left knee, which spread to the right knee, ankles and jaw. Six months later, at the time of the report, arthritis still persisted in her knee (Gross *et al.*, 1994). A 20-year-old woman experienced pain and swelling of her right wrist and fingers 4 days after a hepatitis vaccination. The pain and swelling resolved, but returned again 6 months later with more severe swelling and pain, following a second hepatitis vaccination. Nine years later, X-ray of the hands showed erosive destruction throughout her wrist joints (Gross *et al.*, 1994). A 19-year-old man developed sudden left-ankle arthritis 2 weeks after receiving HBV. Symptoms resolved until he received a second HBV dose and developed swelling of his right knee and left ankle. On blood tests, HLA-B27 antigen was found, which confirmed his diagnosis of reactive arthritis (Hachulla *et al.*, 1990). A 49-year-old woman developed arthritis of her hands within 24 hours of her first HBV vaccination. Her symptoms progressed, with pain and stiffness of wrists, hands, and ankles. Blood tests revealed an elevated RF (rheumatic factor) titre, confirming her diagnosis of rheumatoid arthritis (Vautier & Carty, 1994). Despite the large number of cases submitted to the Vaccine Safety Committee, they refuse to acknowledge that HBV vaccination causes arthritis.

Eighteen cases of **anaphylaxis** were reported in VAERS between 1990 and 1992. Five of these were well-documented reactions that met the Vaccine Safety Committee's strict definitions of anaphylaxis. Others included "anaphylactic-type reactions (cardiovascular collapse associated with wheezing)," that either did not occur within 4 hours of vaccination or had no recording of low blood pressure accompanying the report.

Hepatitis B Summary

1. Hepatitis B is primarily a sexually transmitted disease. Other common sources of transmission include exposure to infected blood, injected-drug use, and occupational or household contacts.
2. Infants can contract hepatitis B from their infected mothers.
3. Women can be tested during pregnancy to determine if they are infected, and infants born to infected mothers can receive hepatitis B vaccine and hepatitis immune globulin at birth.
4. The practice of vaccinating all infants for hepatitis B is unnecessary since only those children exposed to infected mothers are at risk. Antibody levels produced by vaccination will probably decline to non-protective levels before children reach the age when they are sexually active or exposed to other risk factors.
5. Hepatitis B vaccine has been associated with severe, debilitating, and life-threatening adverse reactions.

Recommendations

If a child's mother is hepatitis antigen-positive, then parents may choose to give hepatitis vaccine soon after birth, accompanied by hepatitis immune globulin. Other infants do not need protection. Adolescents should be counseled concerning risk factors for hepatitis B, including sexual activity, exposure to blood products, and intravenous-drug use. Adolescents, their parents, and adults can choose whether the risk of acquiring hepatitis B seems greater than the risk of reactions to the vaccine, some of which are known and others possibly yet to be discovered.

Varicella (Chickenpox)

Chickenpox is universally recognized by parents as a mild and benign disease of childhood. Almost all children are infected at some time and develop permanent immunity from the disease. The disease is caused by the varicella-zoster virus, a member of the herpesvirus family.

The symptoms of chickenpox usually include a fever and runny nose, followed by the appearance of the typical eruptions. These are small, flat, pink areas which soon fill with a clear fluid, and then open and crust over within 2–3 days. They appear in crops, and persist as active lesions for a week. During this time children are usually uncomfortable and itching, especially if they have many eruptions or if these occur on mucus membranes. The disease usually ends uneventfully after a week.

Treatment is directed at making children comfortable. Homeopathic treatment may be helpful for the itching and other bothersome symptoms. Allopathic treatment consists of acyclovir, an antiviral drug. One study found that children treated with acyclovir had fewer skin lesions (average 294 versus 347 in the placebo group) and had fever for a day or two less than the placebo group (Dunkle et al., 1991). Another study found a similar reduction in skin lesions, but no reduction in complication rates or transmission rates to other children (Balfour et al., 1990). These are modest gains for an expensive drug that has its own set of associated adverse effects. It is esti-

mated that treating 4 million children with chickenpox per year in
the United States with acyclovir would cost $128 million each year
(Preblud, 1986).

Disease Complications

Complications of chickenpox include secondary infections of the
skin and neurologic disease. Encephalitis occurs infrequently in children—once in every 4,000 to 10,000 chickenpox cases. Many of these
cases are mild, and hospitalization is required once in every 10,000
to 15,000 cases (Guess *et al.*, 1986). The incidence of encephalitis
and associated deaths has been decreasing. An average of 58 cases of
encephalitis per year was reported between 1972 and 1979. This was
reduced to an average of only 28 cases reported between 1980 and
1983 (Preblud, 1986). Reye syndrome, a dangerous encephalopathy
characterized by convulsions and coma, is another rare complication of chickenpox, and its incidence has also declined dramatically in recent years. The recent avoidance of aspirin during chickenpox
illnesses may be responsible for the reduction in Reye syndrome.

Deaths from chickenpox complications occur in less than 50 children per year. The risk of death from chickenpox in healthy children
is 0.0014 percent (Preblud, 1986). Children with a disease that com-
promises the immune system are more likely to develop complications from chickenpox. These children include cancer and leukemia
patients undergoing chemotherapy, and those with inborn immune
deficiencies, but the vaccine is contraindicated in these children
(Committee, 1995).

With the advent of a vaccine for chickenpox, vaccine experts
have attempted to maximize the emphasis on disease complications
in order to convince doctors that mass vaccination is worthwhile. A
particularly heinous tactic of vaccine-industry rhetoric is the omis-
sion of incidence rates of complications, which tends to distort the
medical view of a disease and overemphasize its seriousness. For
example, contemplate the eye-opening title of one recent review of
chickenpox in the *New England Journal of Medicine,* "Varicella and
herpes zoster: changing concepts of the natural history, control, and
importance of a not-so-benign virus" (Weller, 1983). In another review
published in the *Journal of Infectious Diseases* researchers note,

"Varicella is not necessarily benign even in healthy children. . . . The records of 96 children hospitalized for varicella [found] that 81 were immunologically normal" (Gershon *et al.*, 1992). They neglect to inform readers in that article that only one in every 10,000 to 15,000 cases of chickenpox requires hospitalization.

Adults who contract chickenpox generally have a more prolonged and serious illness. The complication rate is also higher in adults than in children. A severe form of encephalitis occurs more commonly in adults. This diffuse encephalitis is associated with a high mortality rate (5 to 35 percent). Women who contract chickenpox during the first 16 weeks of pregnancy may have children with congenital malformations. The estimated risk in one study of 150 women infected during pregnancy was less than 1 percent (Siegel *et al.*, 1966). Babies who are born within five days of their mother contracting chickenpox have a high risk of death. Severe illness often occurs in these babies during the first five to ten days after birth. The risk of death is estimated at 31 percent (Meyers, 1974).

Varicella Vaccine

The foisting of the chickenpox vaccine on the American public qualifies as one of the great marketing scams of the century. The idea of preventing chickenpox in healthy children is ludicrous to the point of insanity. The selling of this vaccine to the American public could only be due to an unequivocal belief that any vaccine is worthwhile, or the outright avarice of the pharmaceutical industry. After all, as reported in *The Wall Street Journal,* Merck invested over $5 million in chickenpox vaccine development. Their sentiments are aptly expressed by Samuel Katz, Duke University's pediatrics chairman and head of a vaccine panel at the National Academy of Sciences: "Merck isn't going to make back its investment in that vaccine by just distributing it to kids with cancer. They're going to be interested in pushing for use in the normal population" (Wessel, 1985).

The most frequently stated purpose of the chickenpox vaccine is not to protect children from this benign childhood illness, but to keep parents at their jobs rather than missing a few days of work to care for their sick child at home. According to a leading varicella vaccine researcher, "It is clear that we can reduce the cost of chickenpox by routinely immunizing normal children, primarily by reducing the loss of parental income" (Brunell, 1991). Vaccination of the entire population will save an estimated $380 million dollars in lost income and wages (Preblud, 1986). Parents lose 0.5 to 1.8 days of work outside the home while caring for their child with chickenpox (Sullivan-Bolyai *et al.*, 1987). The population is being subjected to this mass experiment, risking the potential long-term adverse effects of the vaccine, so that parents can avoid missing an average of 1 day of work. Economic interests have spurred the adoption of a chickenpox vaccine, not our concern for the well-being of children. This travesty is being perpetrated in the name of public health.

The varicella vaccine was developed in the 1970s, and licensed for children 12 months or older in 1995. Recent studies have evaluated the use of the vaccine in combination with the measles, mumps and rubella shot (Brunell *et al.*, 1988), and it is now recommended that the 4 vaccines be given simultaneously (Committee, 1995).

Vaccine Efficacy

The vaccine seems to be at least 90 percent effective in producing antibodies to the varicella-zoster virus (Arbeter, 1986). These antibodies persist at protective levels for several years. The persistence of immunity over longer periods has not been determined because the vaccine has not been tested in large enough trials for long enough periods of time. During 8 years of study the rate of varicella after vaccination has averaged from 1 to 3 percent per year, compared to an annual varicella rate of 7 to 8 percent in unvaccinated children (Watson *et al.*, 1993). Although researchers assert that when chickenpox occurs in children previously vaccinated their cases are usually mild (Gershon, 1992), a 3.5-year-old boy who had previously developed protective levels of antibodies in response to varicella vaccine contracted chickenpox and aseptic meningitis 21 months later (Naruse *et al.*, 1993). This was the first reported case of such a dramatic vaccine failure.

We can predict the results of mass chickenpox vaccine usage from our experience with measles and mumps vaccines. Just as those diseases have become increasingly more prevalent in adults compared to children, with more likelihood of serious disease and resulting complications, so we are likely to see chickenpox become more common in adults. Persistence of vaccine effectiveness may decline over time. Unusual cases of varicella-zoster illness may also occur, as they do after measles and mumps vaccine. These possible effects are unknown, but they do concern vaccine researchers. Dr. Philip Brunell, in his introduction to a state-of-the-art report on varicella vaccine, describes the reluctance to use the vaccine in normal children because "chickenpox, which is relatively mild in childhood, might increase in frequency during adult life when it is much more severe" (Brunell, 1986). He later stated, "Our present performance in immunizing adults is not good. If we were to find that the protection conferred by varicella vaccine was not durable, re-immunization to prevent chickenpox in adults would be an unreliable solution" (Brunell, 1991). The experience with measles and mumps would seem to justify this cautionary note. Another vaccine researcher stated this concern in even stronger terms:

> One would not, however, want to vaccinate against varicella routinely in childhood if immunity wanes and thereby creates a population of varicella-susceptible adults.... Practically, however, the only means to determine whether waning immunity will be a problem is to vaccinate a large number of healthy children and follow them for many years. Therefore, only post-licensure surveillance of vaccinated children can be utilized to determine if this will be a significant problem (Gershon, 1987).

The vaccine industry is now conducting this colossal experiment.

Vaccine Reactions

Reactions to the vaccine in limited studies have been relatively mild; however, vaccines are usually considered safe initially, and severe reactions are only reported after mass campaigns have vaccinated enough people to generate significant numbers to accumulate statistics. Reports of adverse reactions trickle in slowly. The most common reaction has been a generalized **rash** that resembles naturally acquired chickenpox. This eruption occurs in at least 5 to 10 percent of vaccinees (Arbeter, 1986). Such eruptions have spread to susceptible contacts of vaccinees. In studies of vaccinated children with leukemia, 2 to 10 percent of siblings developed varicella vaccine virus eruptions (Gershon, 1984; Gershon, 1986). No severe adverse reactions have been reported in the studies done so far.

Two possible long-term effects of the vaccine are feared by researchers—herpes zoster and cancer. Varicella-zoster virus can be stored in nerve cells after natural chickenpox infection, and cause a recurrence of infection sometime later in the person's life. This subsequent infection is known as **herpes zoster** or **shingles.** It consists of a very painful skin eruption (the Danish term is "Hell's fire") which may persist for several weeks. Varicella vaccine has caused zoster in normal children (Plotkin, 1988). In one study, 8 of 9,000 healthy children developed zoster subsequent to vaccination (Mangano & White, 1992). The rate of incidence is unknown, and it may or may not be greater than zoster that follows naturally acquired chickenpox.

No one knows the possible effects of latent vaccine virus stored within the nervous system. Varicella-zoster virus may be a cause of **cancer.** This association has never been proven, though varicella-zoster-infected human cells have transformed mouse cells to cancerous cells in a laboratory setting (Yamanishi *et al.,* 1981) and varicella-zoster virus infected cells produced cancers when inoculated into hamsters, which also developed viral antibodies (Gelb *et al.,* 1980). Such findings have led reviewers to comment, "Although no clinical association between the virus and cancer in human beings has even been suggested, the remote possibility of such a relation should be considered in planning long-term surveillance of trials of live-virus vaccines" (Weller, 1983). The possible long-term effects of this herpesvirus vaccine remain unknown.

Mass vaccination of children will be a monumental experiment. Once again, we are injecting children with a live virus which can cause encephalitis and has the ability to remain latent for an entire lifetime. This experiment is being conducted on your children, and the proposed goal is saving money.

Varicella (Chickenpox) Summary

1. Chickenpox is a mild disease of childhood; complications of the disease are rare in healthy children.
2. Adults almost always have more severe infection than children, and disease complications are more common.
3. Long-term efficacy of the vaccine is unknown. Widespread vaccine usage may shift the age distribution of chickenpox from children to adults.
4. Adverse and long-term effects of the vaccine are unknown. They could be more serious than measles and mumps vaccines, because the chickenpox virus is associated with cancer and herpes zoster.

Recommendations

Varicella vaccine has questionable usefulness, and introduces a persisting live virus into the body, which has unknown long-term adverse effects. I do not recommend its use in healthy children because of these uncertainties. Tampering with the immune system in order to save parents' and the corporate world's time and money is patently ridiculous. This is another instance of the vaccine industry's desire to sell a product that we do not need.

Pneumococcal Vaccine

S treptococcus pneumonia (pneumococcus) is a bacterium associated with many cases of pneumonia, meningitis, bacteremia (systemic infection in the bloodstream), and ear infections. At least 10 to 25 percent of all pneumonias culture *S pneumonia* (Williams *et al.*, 1988) and approximately one-third of all ear infections in children are associated with *S pneumonia* growth (Bluestone and Klein, 1988). In addition, the estimated incidence of pneumococcal meningitis is 1 or 2 per 100,000 persons, and pneumococcal bacteremia (infection in the bloodstream) may occur as often as 160 per 100,000 for children under two years of age (Centers for Disease Control, 1989h). The frequent encounters with pneumococcal disease have spurred a search for an effective vaccine. The bacterium has also become increasingly resistant to antibiotics, and this has further stimulated vaccine research.

Several pneumococcal vaccines are under investigation. In 1977, a pneumococcal vaccine was licensed which contained 14 types of *S pneumonia*. This was replaced by a vaccine of 23 types in 1983. These early polysaccharide vaccines have met with limited success, and new vaccine technology is under investigation in which the polysaccharide is bonded to a protein carrier to produce a conjugate vaccine that researchers hope will be more successful.

Undoubtedly, this new vaccine will be included in the growing list of routine vaccinations. Children will probably one day routinely receive the DTP-HIB-HepB-E-IPV-MMRV and PPP (Protein-Polysac-charide Pneumococcal) shot. This is not just a fantasy. Experts in vaccine research have stated, "It is conceivable that within a few years polysaccharide conjugate vaccines including four or more pneu-mococcal types, *H. influenzae* type b, and one or more meningococ-cal groups will be administered with diphtheria and tetanus toxoid and pertussis vaccine to children as young as two months of age" (Bluestone and Klein, 1988, p. 194).

The estimated effectiveness of the pneumococcal vaccine is 60 to 70 percent (Centers for Disease Control, 1989h). However, three studies found little or no effect from the vaccine (Austrian, 1981; Simberkoff *et al.*, 1986; Forrester *et al.*, 1987). Most of the studies have been conducted in high-risk adult patients who are most sus-ceptible to pneumonia. Studies of children reveal that the currently licensed polysaccharide vaccine is ineffective in children under 2 years of age.

Investigations of the pneumococcal vaccine for prevention of ear infections were begun in 1975. Results of three studies showed that vaccinated children had significantly fewer episodes of ear infec-tions associated with the types of *S pneumonia* present in the vac-cine. But children in the vaccine and control groups had the same number of ear infections. In other words, the vaccine did not pre-vent ear infections; it only altered the types of microbes present in the ear (Karma *et al.*, 1980; Makela, *et al.*, 1980, 1981; Sloyer *et al.*, 1981; Teele *et al.*, 1981). The vaccine currently is not recommended for prevention of ear infections.

The only children who now routinely receive the pneumococ-cal vaccine are those at increased risk of serious pneumococcal infec-tions. This group includes those children with certain chronic diseases that impair the immune system, and those who have had their spleen removed (Centers for Disease Control, 1989h).

The vaccine has been associated with few adverse effects. Approx-imately 50 percent of vaccinees (30 to 40 percent in children) devel-op swelling and pain at the injection site. Fever, muscle pain, and severe swelling occur in less than one percent of those vaccinated. High fevers (over 102°) and severe allergic reactions have been report-ed (Committee on Infectious Diseases, 1985).

Pneumococcal Vaccine Summary

1. *Streptococcus pneumonia* is associated with a large percentage of ear infections, meningitis, pneumonia, and bacteremia in children.
2. The currently licensed vaccine is 60 to 70 percent effective in preventing serious disease.
3. Studies do not show any appreciable effect on reduction of ear infections in children.
4. The vaccine is currently recommended for children with chronic diseases, and not for healthy children.

Recommendations

Soon the pneumococcal vaccine will be available for all children. It will be deemed safe and effective in preventing pneumonia, meningitis, and ear infections. It will probably be combined with other vaccines as part of the recommended vaccination schedule. This will occur regardless of its low rate of effectiveness.

The long-term effects of the pneumococcal vaccine are unknown. They will only be discovered if severe reactions occur soon after injection. Otherwise, the effects of this vaccine will be inextricably combined with those of other routine vaccinations of childhood, and we will never know whether there are deleterious effects or not. The same possibilities exist for this vaccine as with the other bacteria and viruses that have neurotoxic effects (pertussis, *Haemophilus*, measles). They all could cause encephalitis and contribute to the brain injury syndrome postulated by Coulter. I cannot recommend this vaccine for healthy children.

New Vaccines

The medical profession and drug manufacturers continually develop new vaccines for childhood illnesses. Research studies are done and cost analyses determine whether the price of the vaccine is worth the prevention of disease and the risk of adverse effects. Debate on this subject occurs, and the FDA eventually decides to license the new vaccine for widespread use. Only then will the millions of dollars invested by drug companies in research and development be recouped many times over in the form of profits.

After a period of time during which large numbers of children are vaccinated, the adverse effects of each vaccine begin to appear. Hundreds of thousands of children must be vaccinated before these adverse effects appear, because vaccine reactions often go unreported, and it is often difficult to attribute delayed effects to a vaccine. The use of new vaccines is an experiment conducted on healthy children.

No research is done on the long-term effects of vaccines before licensure, because drug companies must market their product as quickly as possible. They cannot wait for a thirty-year study. Furthermore, they have little motivation to discover adverse effects or generate negative data about their vaccines. Studies to monitor the adverse effects of vaccines are unpopular, and researchers find it difficult to obtain funding for such projects.

The impetus to discover adverse effects comes from parents of vaccine-injured children and journalists sympathetic to their stories.

The medical profession is quick to adopt new vaccines, and is generally disinterested in their problems. Foot-dragging, delayed responses to problems with vaccines, and suppression of information are the typical official responses by the medical profession when questions of vaccine safety arise.

This course of events has been well-documented in Coulter and Fisher's exposé of the pertussis-vaccine catastrophe (Coulter and Fisher, 1991). The United States Government was compelled to step in and rescue drug companies from the ruinous lawsuits brought against them by dismayed and angry parents of children damaged by the pertussis vaccine. Financial investments of drug companies and the vaccine industry dictate the direction of research on vaccination policy. Their interests lie in promotion of vaccines, not investigation of vaccine reactions.

Despite the history of serious vaccine adverse effects, including polio caused by the oral vaccine, deaths and brain damage caused by DTP, and the many problems of live measles and mumps vaccines, drug companies and the medical profession persist in the development and rush to market of new vaccines. Few studies and little experience precede licensure of these new products. *Haemophilus*, chickenpox, and pneumococcal vaccines are the most recent experiments conducted on America's children.

Conclusion

Most parents take the issue of vaccinations for granted. The pediatrician says their children need them, so they comply. Parents may have misgivings and they may not like the idea, but they often have no support for these feelings. The pediatrician has a powerful influence on parents, and most pediatricians are committed to the campaign for universal vaccination. But questions about vaccination are far from completely answered. Questions of efficacy, risks, and long-term effects remain troubling issues for vaccine researchers.

Some parents are philosophically opposed to the concept of vaccinating their children. They are more horrified by the idea of injecting poisonous substances into their child than they are concerned about the remote future possibility of the diseases. For these parents, the vaccines represent a dangerous form of Russian roulette they are unwilling to play.

Other parents may be anxious about the effects of vaccines on their child, but they are concerned that if enough people avoid the shots then the diseases will begin to reappear: "The vaccines may cause bad reactions, but if I avoid them for my child, then the vaccine campaign will not work for the general population." This is a sacrificial philosophy: "Risk the side effects in my child for the good of the whole society." The stakes of this game may be exceedingly high if the vaccines are capable of causing a covert encephalitis syndrome that potentially affects the whole population. If that is true, then we are trading acute diseases for chronic brain injury. This sacrifice is hardly worth the cost.

I assume that most parents who have read this book are concerned about the adverse effects of vaccines. Most parents are also anxious about some of the diseases discussed here. In fact, for parents, the impetus to give vaccines is primarily based on anxiety: "What if one of these diseases should happen to my unvaccinated child?" The potential guilt factor is tremendous. Never mind that some of the vaccines themselves have very questionable efficacy. If parents do vaccinate, at least they eliminate the guilt if a child contracts a disease. So one of the main tasks for parents to accomplish when they choose not to vaccinate is overcoming anxiety and guilt. But imagine the guilt and self-reproach if your child is severely damaged by a vaccine.

Anxiety about disease is a serious issue for parents. Tetanus is the best example. Parents who choose not to get tetanus shots for their children often think about cuts and puncture wounds. When little Josh climbs up the slide, they wonder about tetanus bacteria in the fertilized soil of the playground. This is enough to distract a parent from enjoying playtime.

Exposure to other children may cause anxiety for parents of unvaccinated children for two reasons. First, you may worry that your child could be exposed to children who bring diseases from other countries. Parents especially worry about polio and whooping cough. Parents should keep in mind the figures cited in the polio section of this book. No cases of polio—except those contracted from the vaccine itself—have occurred in the United States since 1979. This includes immigrants, aliens, and visitors from other countries.

Your child cannot contract a disease unless he or she is exposed to one. Other diseases, such as measles, mumps, and chickenpox do exist in the United States, but exposure to them may be beneficial to your child, providing lifelong immunity. The pertussis vaccine, in my opinion, has too many associated adverse effects to risk its use in any child, regardless of exposure to the disease.

The second anxiety about your unvaccinated child's exposure to others concerns polio. Children who are vaccinated early in life with the oral, live vaccine may shed the virus in their stools. Exposure of your child to recently vaccinated children is a potential hazard, although a small child's exposure to soiled diapers seems highly unlikely. Parents should keep in mind that more than 95 percent of polio illness manifests as a cold. Nonetheless, the risk is there. Parents should be vocal about their concerns. Ask whether playmates and other children in day care have recently received the oral polio vaccine, as opposed to the killed (injected) vaccine which cannot spread the disease. It is appropriate for other parents to be concerned that their vaccinated children could spread the disease to others. They should be educated about this possibility, and assume responsibility for limiting the likelihood of their child spreading the virus to unvaccinated children. In the future, the risk of this exposure will disappear if babies are vaccinated with the killed (E-IPV) polio vaccine, which does not cause polio in recipients or contacts.

The only way for parents of unvaccinated children to feel secure is to remember the original reasons for their decision. Parents often need booster doses of vaccine education. They should keep in mind four points of information:

1. Vaccines cause immediate, sometimes drastic, adverse reactions.
2. Vaccines have unknown long-term adverse effects which may include post-encephalitis brain damage.
3. Vaccine efficacy may decrease over time, making children susceptible to the viral diseases as adults, when the diseases are more serious.
4. Many vaccines are questionably effective.

Parents of unvaccinated children should expect that they will be continually harassed and reproached about their child's "immunization status." Kindred friends may offer support, but the concerns of family members themselves can be almost overwhelming. Grandparents are notorious worriers. Their well-intentioned concern should be politely ignored. At best, parents can offer books like this one, or those in the Resources section, to troubled family members.

If two spouses disagree about vaccination and reach an impasse, then I recommend that the spouse opposed to the vaccines firmly hold his or her ground. There is no more tenacious an animal than a mother protecting her child from harm! If you are convinced that vaccines present a significant threat to your child's health, then do not allow them. No one can inject vaccines without your consent. Withhold your consent if you have serious doubts about their safety and advisability, and seek legal advice if your rights as a parent to refuse vaccines are threatened.

Schools may provide a continual source of difficulty to parents of unvaccinated children. Again, parents should simply hold firm in their resolve. Seek out a medical provider who is willing to sign a medical release. School-district personnel in states that offer a religious or philosophical exemption may need to be educated about this option. Provide them with information about your state's laws governing immunization exemptions. You will be paving the way for another parent in your position. Colleges and universities also require vaccinations, and the same rules apply as for other schools. No child should be vaccinated against a parent's better judgment. Legal protection is available against forced vaccination.

The final frontier in communicating your decision about vaccinations is the pediatrician or family physician. These doctors care for your child, medically and emotionally. They should be a source of support for you and your child. They may disagree with your decision and voice their concerns, but they should respect your opinions and judgments. Talk with them about your concerns, and show them that you are knowledgeable about vaccine reactions and disease incidence. Share this book with them. Do your part in communicating. They will benefit from your insights. If you meet with hostility or terminal resistance, then you may want to seek another medical provider who is more receptive and understanding. Do not give up, and do not be intimidated. Your physician is working for you, as part of a team that cares for your child. And you are the manager of that team.

You will not convince your pediatrician that the entire vaccine industry is wrong. No professional likes to think that their entire training and literature is biased and manipulated for profits by corporations with little concern for altruistic issues. Most pediatricians have the best interests of children at heart. They are convinced that vaccines have saved countless children's lives. They have been trained to accept and praise vaccinations as the most successful preventive intervention in the history of medicine. They are dedicated to continuing this proud tradition of preventive medicine for children.

If you have made an educated and informed decision not to vaccinate your child, then you can be proud of your choice. Remember that doubts often plague parents who choose to vaccinate. They wonder if they did the right thing. Should they continue with boosters once they have started? All those earlier shots might be wasted. If you have doubts at any point, you can stop giving the vaccines. Remember that vaccines often cause severe reactions after the third or fourth shot, even if the first two were well-tolerated.

The doubts of parents with unvaccinated children are even stronger: "Am I risking my child's life when he or she is exposed to strangers or children from 'other cultures' playing in the park?" Parents can never be sure they are doing the right thing. But if your doubts about the safety of the vaccine campaign are strong enough, then it makes sense to allow your child's body to fight off diseases and develop a strong immune system capable of handling infectious disease on its own. This may be one of the greatest gifts you give to your child.

Vaccination Schedules

The following schedules for vaccination have been included so that parents will know what to expect from health providers who recommend the vaccines. Vaccinations can be delayed and given at any time parents prefer. Parents can choose to give some vaccines and not others. If you decide to give the vaccines, the tetanus, diphtheria, pertussis, or polio vaccines should be given as a series, in order to achieve recommended antibody levels. The combined vaccines, with *Haemophilus,* diphtheria, tetanus, pertussis, and inactivated polio, can each be given alone.

Recommended Vaccination Schedule for Infants from Birth

Vaccine	Birth	1–2 mos	2 mos	4 mos	6 mos	6–18 mos	12–15 mos	15 mos	4–6 yrs
Diphtheria-tetanus-pertussis			DTP	DTP	DTP			DTP/DTaP	DTP/DTaP
Polio, live oral (option)			OPV IPV	OPV IPV	OPV			OPV	OPV OPV
Measles-mumps-rubella							MMR		MMR*
Haemophilus influenzae b conjugate			Hib	Hib	Hib		Hib		
Hepatitis B (optional schedule)	HepB	HepB HepB		HepB	HepB	HepB			
Varicella-zoster virus (chicken-pox)							VZV		VZV

*can be administered at 12–13 years old

Recommended Vaccination Schedule
for Children up to 7 Years Old

First visit	DTP, OPV, Hib MMR, VZV (if > 12 mos)
1 month later	DTP, Hib, HepB
2 mos later	DTP, OPV, Hib
3 mos later	OPV
9 mos later	DTP/DTaP, Hib, HepB
At 4–6 yrs old	Td, OPV, MMR, VZV

Note: For children beginning the series after 7 years of age the schedule is
similar, but Td (tetanus and diphtheria toxoid) is substituted for DTP

Resources

Organizations

National Vaccine Information Center (NVIC)
operated by Dissatisfied Parents Together (DPT)
    512 W. Maple Avenue, #206
    Vienna, VA 22180
    800–909–SHOT
    703–938–DPT3
    FAX 703–938–5768

An organization of concerned lay people and professionals that promotes information about vaccines, promotes legislation relating to safe vaccinations and free choice, and assists parents in their legal battles to obtain compensation for vaccine injury, to avoid vaccination in situations where legal pressures are applied. Members receive a regular newsletter. They publish a law-firm directory, and booklets on the vaccine-injury compensation system and instructions for filing claims.

Centers for Disease Control
  National Immunization Program
  Information Services Office
  Mail Stop E-06
  Atlanta, GA 30333–4018
  800–232–SHOT
  International Travelers Hotline
  404–332–4559

Provides information to the public on vaccination policies,
standards, and recommendations, as well as international travel
and disease outbreaks around the world.

National Center for Homeopathy
  801 North Fairfax St., Suite 306
  Alexandria, VA 22314
  703–548–7790

Information resource center for homeopathic medicine. They publish a national directory of homeopathic practitioners.

Council for Homeopathic Certification
  P.O. Box 157
  Corte Madera, CA 94976
  415–389–9502

A certification board that tests practitioners in classical
homeopathy through a written and oral examination—voluntary
certification that assures consumers that practitioners are well-
qualified in homeopathic principles and practice. They publish a
directory of certificate holders.

Homeopathic Educational Services
  2124 Kittredge St.
  Berkeley, CA 94704
  800–359–9051 (orders)
  510–649–0294
  FAX 510–649–1955

A distributor and mail-order supplier of homeopathic books, medicines, audiotapes and summaries of homeopathic research. Send
for extensive catalog.

Vaccine Adverse Event Reporting System
P.O. Box 1100
Rockville, MD 20849–1100
800–822–7967

The surveillance system established by the National Childhood Vaccine Injury Act to collect reports of adverse reactions following vaccination. Health care providers are obligated to report specific adverse events following particular vaccines. Parents, other relatives or anyone aware of the occurrence of an adverse event may also file a report. Call for reporting forms.

Legal Resources

Immunization Hotline
James Filenbaum
2 Executive Blvd. #201–P
Suffern, NY 10901
800–753–LAWS
914–357–0020

A law firm specializing in vaccination law and exemptions. They assist parents in securing religious exemptions based on individual religious belief. Representation for parents seeking compensation for vaccine damage.

National Vaccine Information Center (NVIC)
Operated by Dissatisfied Parents Together (DPT)
512 W. Maple Avenue, #206
Vienna, VA 22180
800–909–SHOT
703–938–DPT3
FAX 703–938–5768

They publish a law firm directory, and booklets on the vaccine injury compensation system and instructions for filing claims.

Publications

The Immunization Resource Guide, by Diane Rozario
Patter Publications
P.O. Box 204
Burlington, IA 52601

The most complete single resource for books, organizations, information services, publishers, and government offices that have anything to do with vaccines, both pro and con. Extensive annotated bibliography, address lists, book reviews, and organization descriptions. The complete directory on vaccination for the consumer.

New Atlantean Press
P.O. Box 9638
Santa Fe, NM 87504
505–983–1856

Mail order supplier of vaccination books and other health related topics. They stock virtually every book critical of vaccines.

International Vaccination Newsletter
c/o Kris Baubloumme, M.D.
Krekenstrasat 4, Genk N-3600, Belgium
Tel: 011–32–11–227869
FAX: 011–32–89–304982

Quarterly publication from Europe, provides information about vaccinations, linking organizations throughout the world in the vaccine field.

Books

Coulter, H.L. *Vaccination, Social Violence, and Criminality: The Medical Assault on the American Brain,* North Atlantic Books, Berkeley, California, 1990.

Describes childhood immunizations as a possible cause of encephalitis characterized by learning problems, developmental delays, behavior disorders, and autism.

Coulter, H.L. & Fisher, B.L. *A Shot in the Dark,* Avery Publishing
Group, Inc., Garden City, New York, 1991.

Documentation of the devastating effects of the pertussis vaccine,
including vivid case examples and an exposé of the campaign for
mandatory immunization of children regardless of the risks.

Cummings, S. & Ullman, D. *Everybody's Guide to Homeopathic Medicines,* Jeremy P Tarcher/Putnam, New York, 1991.

An introduction to homeopathic principles, and the use of
homeopathic medicines to treat common acute illnesses of
children and adults.

James, W. *Immunization: The Reality Behind the Myth,* Bergin &
Garvey Publishers, Granberry, Massachusetts, 1995.

A description of the problems with immunization statistics and a
proposal for parents to build a strong immune system in their children without using vaccines.

Mendelsohn, R. *How to Raise a Healthy Child ... In Spite of Your
Doctor,* Contemporary Books, Chicago, 1984.

A practical and common-sense guide advising parents to avoid
overtreatment, immunizations and other hazards encountered in
the pediatrician's office.

Miller, N. *Vaccines: Are They Really Safe and Effective?* New
Atlantean Press, Santa Fe, 1992; and *Immunization: Theory vs.
Reality,* New Atlantean Press, Santa Fe, 1996.

Both books take a hard-hitting critical approach to vaccinations.
Vaccines presents the issues surrounding each vaccine in summary
form. *Immunization* provides detailed descriptions of the vaccine
industry's tactics: threats, evasion, denial, and genocidal policies.

Murphy, J. *What Every Parent Should Know about Childhood
Immunization,* Earth Healing Products, Boston, 1993.

A thorough and easily understandable critique of vaccination
based on arguments about toxicity, low efficacy, and failure to
establish true immunity to disease.

Reprints of articles

Richard Moskowitz, MD, *The Case Against Immunizations*

A fascinating theoretical investigation of vaccine adverse effects, with emphasis on their possible role in immune system dysfunction. Fairly technical.

> National Center for Homeopathy
> 801 North Fairfax St., Suite 306
> Alexandria, VA 22314
> 703–548–7790

Vaccinations: The Rest of the Story

A collection of articles from Mothering, reprinted in booklet form. These give a wide-ranging view, including articles by physicians and parents about many areas of concern to parents who must make the immunization decision.

> *Mothering Magazine*
> P.O. Box 1690
> Santa Fe, NM 87504
> 505–984–8116

Vaccine Information Websites on the Internet

(All addresses preeded by http://www.)

The following sites provide links to most major vaccine information resources on the Internet.

healthy.net/vaccine

Vaccination resources, articles, and current information from Randall Neustaedter within the HealthWorld alternative medicine website. Dr. Neustaedter conducts a forum for the public, answering questions about vaccines and vaccine choices.

access1.net/via

Vaccine Information & Awareness (VIA) contains links to most other websites with vaccine information, including both pro-vaccine and pro-choice sites. All the facts about vaccines online that anyone could want. Karin Schumacher compiles data on a daily basis and supplies articles through her news service. Contact her at via@access1.net to receive postings by e-mail. Beware though, the mail service is for people with a serious interest in vaccine information˜voluminous materials culled from the medical literature.

909shot.com

Website for the National Vaccine Information Center, a parent-sponsored group which lobbies for safer vaccines and freedom of choice legislation. The site includes their newsletter, referral information, and the ability to order books and materials from their extensive catalog.

thinktwice.com

This site, run by Neil Z. Miller, the author of several popular books about vaccines contains ordering information for books on vaccines and other health related topics. The site also contains articles about vaccines and an inclusive list of worldwide vaccination support groups, legal resources, and information services.

i-wayco.com/niin/index.html

Natural Immunity Information Network, directed by Jessica Hall, contains resources, news and general information for parents about vaccines.

The author can be reached for questions about vaccination on his internet forum at

http://www.healthy.net/vaccine

Glossary

acellular pertussis vaccine—A vaccine prepared from one or more antigens derived from the active components of the *B pertussis* bacterium, particularly pertussis toxin. Developed in an attempt to reduce the adverse effects associated with the whole cell pertussis vaccine.

acupuncture—A technique involving the insertion of fine stainless steel needles into points on the surface of the body that trigger healing responses. Administered in accordance with the theories and principles of Chinese medicine.

adjuvant—A chemical, such as aluminum, added to vaccines to promote antibody response and increase the effectiveness of vaccines.

adsorb—To bind one substance, through a chemical process, to the surface molecule of another in order to promote or increase its effectiveness.

AIDS—Acquired Immunodeficiency Syndrome, a disease characterized by failure of the immune system and accompanied by opportunistic infections (e.g., pneumonia and fungal infections), skin cancers, wasting, and death.

anaphylaxis—An acute, often explosive, systemic reaction characterized by skin eruptions including hives and rashes, respiratory distress and cardiac collapse that may prove fatal. It occurs in a previously sensitized person who again receives the sensitizing antigen.

antigen—Allergen; any material (protein, toxoid, microorganism) that can induce a state of sensitivity or resistance in the body to that material when it is encountered again.

antibody—Any body substance manufactured in response to the stimulus of an antigen introduced into the body, that reacts specifically with that antigen. Many antibodies fight infection and indicate immunity to specific diseases.

arthropathy—Any joint disease, often associated with joint swelling and pain.

autoimmune response—An antibody response developed by the body against its own tissues or cells.

carcinogenic—Having the ability, as a chemical or substance, to cause cancer.

case-control study—A controlled observational study that starts with the identification of persons with a disease or condition (adverse event) of interest and a suitable control group of persons without the disease. The relation of an attribute (e.g., vaccination) to the disease is examined by comparing the diseased and nondiseased groups with regard to how frequently the attribute is present.

chronic fatigue syndrome—A condition characterized by persistent tiredness and other symptoms which may include fevers, poor concentration, joint and muscle pain, sore throat, swollen lymph nodes, and headaches, following a sudden onset of symptoms, often flu-like in nature, but continuing into a persistent or relapsing state.

CNS—Central nervous system; the brain and spinal cord.

conjugate—To bind a vaccine to a protein carrier, thereby increasing its efficacy.

dementia—Loss of brain functions that can manifest as loss of memory, learning ability, and motor control.

demyelination—A process in which the myelin sheath, which acts like an insulator on some nerves, is destroyed, resulting in faulty nerve and brain function.

diabetes—Specifically Insulin-Dependent Diabetes Mellitus (IDDM), characterized by an insufficiency of insulin secretion by the pancreas and an inability to metabolize sugars. Diabetes is thought to arise in response to both genetic and environmental factors.

double-blind study—A clinical experiment in which neither the subjects nor the experimenters know which individual subjects receive the active treatment or intervention and which subjects receive a placebo or non-medicinal treatment.

DTP (or DPT)—Diphtheria toxoid, tetanus toxoid, and pertussis vaccine.

EEG—Electroencephalogram; measurement of brainwaves (changes in electrical potential) by means of electrodes attached to the skull, used to diagnose epilepsy and localize brain lesions.

E-IPV—Enhanced Inactivated Polio Vaccine. Produced in human cells rather than monkey cells, this vaccine has a higher antigenic content and can be used in fewer doses than conventional IPV.

encephalitis—An inflammatory response within the brain.

encephalopathy—A clinical condition with a spectrum of characteristics including altered levels of consciousness, confusion, irritability, changes in behavior, screaming attacks, neck stiffness, convulsions, visual, auditory and speech disturbances, and motor and sensory deficit.

epithelial cell—The surface layer covering the skin, mucus membranes, glands, and body cavities.

GBS (Guillain-Barré Syndrome)—A demyelinating inflammatory disease of the peripheral nervous system with rapid onset of motor weakness and loss of sensation.

HBV—Hepatitis B vaccine.

hemolytic anemia—An abnormally low number of red blood cells caused by their destruction.

homeopathy—The practice of prescribing natural substances (plant, mineral, or animal) according to the principle that such a substance can cure the same symptoms that it can cause. When used medicinally, these substances are usually prepared through a process of serial dilution that enhances their ability to stimulate healing responses in the body.

HIV—Human Immunodeficiency Virus; A retrovirus associated with AIDS. HIV-1 is associated with AIDS cases in Europe and the Americas, HIV-2 with African cases.

HTLV—Human T-Lymphotropic Virus; A group of retroviruses that infect humans and cause leukemia and cancer of lymph nodes.

IDDM Insulin-Dependent Diabetes Mellitus—see diabetes.

IgE antibody—One of the immunoglobulins within the blood that denotes allergy to specific antigens. For example, the presence of

IgE antibody to milk within a person's blood shows that an individual has allergic responses to milk.

IPV—Inactivated Polio Vaccine (killed vaccine or Salk vaccine); a sterile suspension of three types of polioviruses used as an injection to vaccinate against polio.

leukemia—A disease characterized by an abnormal continuing increase in white blood cells.

lymphocyte—A white blood cell responsible for providing protection against infection and disease.

meningitis—Inflammation of the membranes of the brain or spinal cord.

MMR—Measles, mumps, and rubella vaccine.

MSAEFI—Monitoring System for Adverse Events Following Immunization; a passive-surveillance system designed and monitored by the Centers for Disease Control for the purpose of collecting nationwide data on adverse events associated with vaccination.

multiple sclerosis—A chronic central nervous system demyelinating disease in which the nerve lesions occur in multiple locations.

myelin—The sheath, on the surface of a nerve, made of fats and protein that acts as an insulator.

neurologic—Pertaining to the nervous system.

optic neuritis—A central demyelinating disease of the optic nerve, affecting vision.

OPV—Oral Polio Vaccine; a live-virus vaccine prepared from three types of poliovirus given as an oral dose.

passive surveillance—The collection of voluntary reports from health care providers and the public that describe adverse vaccine reactions.

potency—The strength of a homeopathic medicine corresponding to the number of times it has been diluted and shaken in the pharmaceutical preparation process. These numbers are typically recorded as 12x, 30x, 30c, 200c, 1M, etc., signifying whether the dilutions occurred 1/10 (x) or 1/100 (c), and the number of dilutions performed.

PRP—The early polysaccharide capsular *Haemophilus influenzae* type b vaccine, which is no longer used. The name "PRP" corresponds to the polysaccharide itself, a repeating polymer of ribose and ribitol linked by a phosphate group.

purpura—Bleeding into the skin, mucus membranes, and internal organs.

relative risk—The ratio of the risk of disease or other outcome among the exposed compared to the risk among the unexposed.

SIDS—Sudden Infant Death Syndrome; the unexpected and unexplained death of an apparently well infant.

SIV—Simian Immunodeficiency Virus; A group of retroviruses found in monkeys that are associated with Simian Acquired Immunodeficiency, (simian AIDS).

squamous cells—Cells in the form of scales that are spread like a pavement over the superficial layer of body cavities or surface membranes.

SSPE—See subacute sclerosing panencephalitis.

STLV—Simian T-Lymphotropic Virus; A group of retroviruses that infect monkeys.

Subacute sclerosing panencephalitis—A form of brain inflammation characterized by insidious onset of a progressive cerebral dysfunction occurring over the course of weeks or months. Symptoms include jerking motions, spasticity, difficulty swallowing, and progressive loss of vision. The average patient dies within 2 years after a persistent coma.

SV-40—The fortieth simian virus discovered.

thrombocytopenia—A decrease in blood platelets responsible for blood clotting with accompanying spontaneous bleeding.

toxoid—The toxin of a microorganism that has been treated (commonly with formaldehyde) to diminish its toxic effects, but which still has the power to stimulate antibody production.

Traditional Chinese Medicine—The science of using herbs, acupuncture and related practices based on principles of healing developed in China over the past 5,000 years.

transverse myelitis—A set of symptoms, including lack of motor control and sensation in isolated parts of the body, suggesting a lesion at one level of the spinal cord.

VAERS—Vaccine Adverse Event Reporting System; a passive surveillance system intended to collect reports of reactions to vaccines operated by the Centers for Disease Control and the U.S. Food and Drug Administration.

VAPP—Vaccine Associated Paralytic Poliomyelitis; polio caused by the vaccine rather than a natural infection.

References

AAP News, Vaccine brochures: AAP proposes changes. June 1989, p. 2.

Aberer, W. Vaccination despite thimerosal sensitivity. *Contact Dermatitis* 1991; 24:6–10.

Abernathy, R.S., Spink, W.W. Increased susceptibility of mice to bacterial endotoxins induced by pertussis vaccine. Fed Proc 1956; 15:580.

ACHA (American College Health Association). Position statement on immunization policy. *Journal of American College Health* 1983; 32:7–8.

Acheson, E.D.; Barnes, H.R.; Gardner, M.J. *et al.* Formaldehyde in the British chemical industry. An occupational cohort study. *Lancet* 1984; 1(8377):611–616.

Ad hoc group for the study of pertussis vaccines. Placebo-controlled trial of two acellular pertussis vaccines in Sweden—Protective efficacy and adverse events. *Lancet* 1988; I:955–960.

Adler, J.B., Mazzotta, S.A., Barkin, J.S. Pancreatitis caused by measles, mumps, and rubella vaccine. *Pancreas* 1991; 6:489–490.

Agy, M.B., Frumkin, L.R., Corey, L. *et al.* Infection of Macaca nemestrina by human immunodeficiency virus type 1. *Science* 1992; 257:103–106.

Albert, R.E., Sellakumar, A.R., Laskin, S. *et al.* Gaseous formaldehyde and hydrogen chloride induction of nasal cancer in the rat. *Journal of the National Cancer Institute* 1982; 68(4):597–603.

Albrecht, P., Ennis, F.A., Saltzman, E.J., Krugman, S. Persistence of maternal antibody in infants beyond 12 months: mechanisms of measles vaccine failure. *Journal of Pediatrics* 1977; 91:715–718.

Alderslade, R., Bellman, M.H., Rawson, N.S. *et al.* The National Childhood Encephalopathy Study, in Whooping Cough: Reports from the Committee on Safety of Medicines and the Joint Committee on Vaccination and Immunisation. London, Department of Health and Social Security, Her Majesty's Stationery Office, 1981, pp 79–154.

Alfrey, A.C. *et al.* Syndrome of dyspraxia and multifocal seizures associated with chronic hemodialysis. *Transactions of the American Society of Artificial Internal Organs* 1972; 18:257.

Alfrey, A.C. *et al.* The dialysis encephalopathy syndrome, possible aluminum intoxication. *New England Journal of Medicine* 1976; 94:184.

Alter, M.J., Hadler, S.C., Margolis, H.S., Alexander J. *et al.* The changing epidemiology of hepatitis B in the United States. *Journal of the American Medical Association* 1990; 263:1218–1222.

American Institute of Homeopathy. Special Report of the Homeopathic Yellow Fever Commission Ordered by the AIH for Presentation to Congress. Philadelphia and New York: Boericke and Tafel, 1880.

Andrus, J.K., Strebel, P.M., de Quadros, C.A., Olivé, J.M. Risk of vaccine-associated paralytic poliomyelitis in Latin America, 1989–91. *Bulletin of the World Health Organization* 1995; 73:33–40.

Arbeter, A.M., Starr, S.E., Plotkin, S.A. Varicella vaccine studies in healthy children and adults. *Pediatrics* 1986; 78 (suppl):748–756.

Aukrust, L., Almeland, T.L., Refsum, D., Aas, K. Severe hypersensitivity or intolerance reactions to measles vaccine in six children: clinical and immunological studies. *Allergy* 1980; 35:581–587.

Austrian, R. *Review Infectious Disease* 1981; 3 (suppl):S1–S17.

Backon, J. Prolonged breast feeding as a prophylaxis for recurrent otitis media: relevance of prostaglandins. *Medical Hypotheses* 1984, 13:161.

Bakir, F., Damluji, S.F., Amin-Zaki, L. *et al.* Methylmercury poisoning in Iraq. *Science* 1973; 181:230–241.

Balfour, H.H., Kelly, J.M., Suarez, C.S. *et al.* Acyclovir treatment of varicella in otherwise healthy children. *Journal of Pediatrics* 1990; 116:633–639.

Ballinger, A.B., Clark, M.L. Severe acute hepatitis B infection after vaccination. *Lancet* 1994; 344:1292–1293.

Bannister, B., and Corbel, M.J. The effect of Schick testing on diphtheria antitoxin status. *Journal of Infection* 1991; 22: 11–15.

Baraff, L.J., Ablon, W.J., Weiss, R.C. Possible temporal association between diphtheria-tetanus toxoid-pertussis vaccination and sudden infant death syndrome. *Pediatric Infectious Diseases* 1983; 2:7–11.

Baraff, L.J., Shields, D., Beckwith, L. *et al.* Infants and children with convulsions and hypotonic-hyporesponsive episodes following diphtheria-tetanus-pertussis immunization: follow-up evaluation. *Pediatrics* 1988; 81:789–794.

Barr, M., Glenny, A.T., Randall, K.J. Concentratioon of diphtheria antitoxin in cord blood. *Lancet* 1949; ii: 324–326.

Barrett, L.J. *et al.* Dialysis-associated dementia. *Australian and New Zealand Journal of Medicine* 1975; 5:62.

Bart, K.J., Orenstein, W.A., Preblud, S.R., Hinman, A.R. Universal immunization to interrupt rubella. *Review of Infectious Diseases* 1985; 7 (suppl 1):S177–184.

Bartos, H.R. Thrombocytopenia asociated with rubella vaccination. *New York State Journal of Medicine* 1972; 72:499.

Bass, J.W. Pertussis: current status of prevention and treatment. *Pediatric Infectious Diseases* 1985; 4:614–619.

Beale, A.J. Measles vaccines. *Proceedings of the Royal Society of Medicine* 1974; 67:1116–1119.

Beall, J.R., Ulsamer, A.G. Formaldehyde and hepatotoxicity: a review. *Journal of Toxicology and Environmental Health* 1984; 14(1):1–21.

Beasley R.P., Hwang, L-Y. Epidemiology of hepatocellular carcinoma. In: Vyas, G.N., Dienstag, J.L., Hoofnagle, J.H., eds. *Viral hepatitis and liver disease.* New York: Grune & Stratton, 1984:209–224.

Berg, J.M. Neurological complications of pertussis immunization. *British Medical Journal* 1958; 2:24–27.

Berkowitz, C.D., Ward, J.I., Meier, K. *et al.* Persistence of antibody (AB) to Haemophilus influenzae type b (Hib) and response to PRP and PRP-D booster immunization in children initially immunized with either vaccine at 15 to 24 months (Abstract no. 889). *Pediatric Research* 1987; 21:321A.

Bernstein, H.H., Rothstein, E.P., Pichichero, M.E. *et al.* Clinical reactions and immunogenicity of the BIKEN acellular diphtheria and tetanus toxoids and pertussis vaccine in 4– through 6–year old US children. *American Journal of Diseases of Children* 1992; 146:556–559.

Black, S., Shinefield, H., Hiatt, R.A. *et al.* b-CAPSA 1 Haemophilus influenzea type b capsular polysaccharide vaccine safety. *Pediatrics* 1987; 79: 321–325.

Black, S., Shinefield, H., Hiatt, R.A. *et al.* Efficacy of *Haemophilus influenzea* type b capsular polysaccharide vaccine *Pediatric Infectious Disease Journal* 1988; 7: 149–156.

Black, S., Shinefield, H., Fireman, B., Hiatt, R. *et al.* Efficacy in infancy of oligosaccharide conjugate *Haemophilus influenzae* type b (HbOC) vaccine in a United States population of 61,080 children. *Pediatric Infectious Disease Journal* 1991; 10:97–104.

Black, S.B., Cherry, J.D., Shinefield, H.R. *et al.* Apparent decreased risk of invasive bacterial disease after heterologous childhood immunization. *American Journal of Diseases of Children* 1991(a); 145: 746–749.

Blair, A.; Stewart, P.; O'Berg, M.;*et al.* Mortality among industrial workers exposed to formaldehyde. *Journal of the National Cancer Institute*, 1986; 76(6):1071–1084.

Blair, A., Saracci, R., Stewart, P.A. *et al.* Epidemiologic evidence on the relationship between formaldehyde exposure and cancer. *Scandinavian Journal of Work, Environment and Health* 1990; 16(6):381–393.

Blennow, M., Granstr^m, M. Adverse reactions and serologic response to a booster dose of acellular pertussis vaccine in children immunized with acellular or whole-cell vaccine as infants. *Pediatrics* 1989; 84:62–67.

Bluestone, C.D., Klein, J.O. *Otitis Media in Infants and Children.* Philadelphia: W.B. Saunders Company, 1988.

Bohannon, R.C., Donehower, L.A., Ford, R.J. Isolation of a Type D retrovirus from B-cell lymphomas of a patient with AIDS. *Journal of Virology* 1991; 65:5663–5672.

Bottiger, M., Christenson, B., Romanus, V. *et al.* Swedish experience of two dose vaccination programme aiming at eliminating measles, mumps, and rubella. *British Medical Journal* 1987; 295:1264–1267.

Bowie, C. Lessons from the pertussis vaccine court trial. *Lancet* 1990; 335:397–399.

Bradford, T.L. *The Logic of Figures or Comparative Results of Homeopathic and Other Treatments.* Philadelphia: Boericke and Tafel, 1900.

Brodsky, L., Stanievich, J. Sensorineural hearing loss following live measles virus vaccination. *International Journal of Pediatric Otorhinolaryngology* 1985; 10:159–163.

Broome, C.V. Epidemiology of *Haemophilus influenzae* type b infections in the United States. *Pediatric Infectious Disease Journal* 1987; 6:779–782.

Brunell, P.A. Varicella vaccine—Where are we? *Pediatrics* 1986; 78 (suppl):721–722.

Brunell, P.A., Novelli, V.M., Lipton, S.V., Pollock, B. Combined vaccine against measles, mumps, rubella, and varicella. *Pediatrics* 1988; 81:779–784.

Brunell, P.A. Chickenpox—examining our options. *New England Journal of Medicine* 1991; 325:1577–1579.

Burnett, J.C. *Vaccinosis and its Cure by Thuja.* 1892, published in *Best of Burnett.* New Delhi, India: B. Jain, 1992.

Byers, R.K., Moll, F.C. Encephalopathies following prophylactic pertussis vaccination. *Pediatrics* 1948; 1:437–457.

California Department of Health Services. Measles in Southeast Asian children in the San Joaquin Valley. *California Morbidity* 1990; 51/52.

California Department of Health Services. DTP Vaccine: Truth and consequences, a two-part series. *California Morbidity* 1994; 1.

California Medical Association. Amicus curiae brief of California Medical Association. People of the State of California v. Donna Shalala *et al.* No. 93–15700 in the United States Court of Appeals for the Ninth Circuit. 1993.

Calman, K.C. Measles vaccination as a risk factor for inflammatory bowel disease (letter). *Lancet* 1995; 345:1362.

Candy, J.M., Oakley, A.E., Klinowski, J. *et al.* Aluminosilicates and senile plaque formation in Alzheimerís disease. *Lancet* 1986; I:354–357.

Castro, D., Nogueira, G.G. Use of the nosode Meningococcinum as a preventive against meningitis. *Journal of the American Institute of Homeopathy* 1975; 68:211–219.

Centers for Disease Control. Mumps Surveillance. *MMWR (Morbidity and Mortality Weekly Report)* 1972; No. 2.

Centers for Disease Control. Tetanus in a child with improper medical exemption from immunization—Florida. *MMWR (Morbidity and Mortality Weekly Report)* 1985; 34: 550–552.

Centers for Disease Control. Tetanus—United States, 1982–1985. *MMWR (Morbidity and Mortality Weekly Report)* 1985; 34: 602, 607–611.

Centers for Disease Control. International notes: Imported paralytic poliomyelitis—United States, 1986. *MMWR (Morbidity and Mortality Weekly Report)* 1986; 35:671–674.

Centers for Disease Control. Tetanus—United States, 1982–1986. *MMWR (Morbidity and Mortality Weekly Report)* 1987; 36:477–481.

Centers for Disease Control. Prevention of *Haemophilus influenzae* type b disease. *MMWR (Morbidity and Mortality Weekly Report)* 1988; 37:13–16.

Centers for Disease Control. Measles—Quebec. *MMWR (Morbidity and Mortality Weekly Report)* 1989(a); 38:329–330.

Centers for Disease Control. ACIP: General recommendation on immunization. *MMWR (Morbidity and Mortality Weekly Report)* 1989(b); 38:205–227.

Centers for Disease Control. Measles—Los Angeles County, California, 1988. *MMWR (Morbidity and Mortality Weekly Report)* 1989(c); 38:49–57.

Centers for Disease Control. ACIP: Measles prevention: supplementary statement. *MMWR (Morbidity and Mortality Weekly Report)* 1989(d); 38:11–14.

Centers for Disease Control. Mumps—United States, 1985–1988. *MMWR (Morbidity and Mortality Weekly Report)* 1989(e); 38:101–105.

Centers for Disease Control. Rubella and congenital rubella syndrome—United States, 1985–1988. *MMWR (Morbidity and Mortality Weekly Report)* 1989(f) 38:173–178.

Centers for Disease Control. Mumps prevention. *MMWR (Morbidity and Mortality Weekly Report)* 1989(g) 38:388–400.

Centers for Disease Control. Pneumococcal polysaccharide vaccine. *MMWR (Morbidity and Mortality Weekly Report)* 1989(h); 38:64–76.

Centers for Disease Control. Measles prevention: recommendation of the Immunization Practices Advisory Committee (ACIP). *MMWR (Morbidity and Mortality Weekly Report)* 1989(i); 38:(No. S-9).

Centers for Disease Control. Pertussis surveillance—United States, 1986–1988. *MMWR (Morbidity and Mortality Weekly Report)* 1990; 39:57–66.

Centers for Disease Control. Measles—United States, 1990. *MMWR (Morbidity and Mortality Weekly Report)* 1991; 40:369–372.

Centers for Disease Control. Update: Eradication of paralytic poliomyelitis in the Americas. *MMWR (Morbidity and Mortality Weekly Report)* 1991(a); 41:681–683.

Centers for Disease Control. Hepatitis B virus: a comprehensive strategy for eliminating transmission in the United States through universal childhood vaccination. Recommendations of the Immunization Practices Advisory Committee (ACIP). *MMWR (Morbidity and Mortality Weekly Report)*, 1991(c); 40, No RR-13.

Centers for Disease Control. Asthma—United States, 1980–1990. *MMWR (Morbidity and Mortality Weekly Report)* 1992, 41:733–735.

Centers for Disease Control. Measles surveillance—United States, 1991. *MMWR (Morbidity and Mortality Weekly Report)* 1992(b), 41: (No. SS-6) 1–13.

Centers for Disease Control. Pertussis vaccination: acellular pertussis vaccine for reinforcing and booster use—Recommendations of the Immunization Practices Advisory Committee (ACIP). *MMWR (Morbidity and Mortality Weekly Report)* 1992(c), 41:(No. RR-1) 1–10.

Centers for Disease Control. Recommendations for use of Haemophilus b conjugate vaccines and a combined diphtheria, tetanus, pertussis, and Haemophilus b vaccine; Recommendations fo the Advisory Committee on Immunization Practices (ACIP). *MMWR (Morbidity and Mortality Weekly Report)*, 1993, 42: No. RR-13.

220   THE VACCINE GUIDE

Centers for Disease Control. Summary of notifiable diseases, United States, 1993. *MMWR (Morbidity and Mortality Weekly Report)* 1994, 42: No. 53.

Centers for Disease Control. Vaccination coverage of 2–year-old children—United States, 1992–1993. *MMWR (Morbidity and Mortality Weekly Report)* 1994(a); 43:282–283.

Centers for Disease Control. Progress toward global eradication of poliomyelitis, 1988–1993. *MMWR (Morbidity and Mortality Weekly Report)* 1994(b); 43:499–503.

Chaffin, D., Dinman, B., Miller, J. *et al.* An evaluation of the effects of chronic mercury exposure on EMG and psychomotor functions. *U.S. Department of Health and Human Services, National Institute of Occupational Safety and Health.* Document no. HSM-099-71-62. Washington, DC, 1973.

Chandra, R.K. Immunological aspects of human milk. *Nutrition Review* 1978; 36:265.

Chantler, J.K., Tingle, A.J., Petty, R.E. Persistent rubella virus infection associated with chronic arthritis in children. *New England Journal of Medicine* 1985; 313:1117.

Chavanon, P. *La Diptherie.* Paris: 1932.

Cherry, J.D. 'Pertussis vaccine encephalopathy': It is time to recognize it as the myth that it is. *Journal of the American Medical Association* 1990; 263:1679–1680.

Cherry, J.D., Feigin, R.D., Lobes, L.A., Shackelford, P.G. Atypical measles in children previously immunized with attenuated measles virus vaccines. *Pediatrics* 1972; 50:712.

Cherry, J.D., Brunell, P.A., Golden, G.S., Karzon, D.T. Report of the task force on pertussis and pertussis immunization—1988. *Pediatrics* 1988; 81 (suppl):939–984.

Cherry, J.D., Baraff, L.J., Hewlett, E. The past, present, and future of pertussis: the role of adults in epidemiology and future control (Specialty Conference). *Western Journal of Medicine* 1989; 150:319–328.

Church, J.A, Richards, W. Recurrent abscess formation following DTP immunizations: association with hypersensitivity to tetanus toxoid. *Pediatrics* 1985; 75:899–900.

Cizman, M., Mozetic, M., Radescek-Rakar, R. *et al.* Aseptic meningi-

tis after vaccination against measles and mumps. *Pediatric Infectious Disease Journal* 1989; 8:302–308.

Clarke, J.H. *A Dictionary of Practical Materia Medica*. Sussex, England: Health Science Press, 1967.

Clemens, J.D., Ferreccio, C., Levine, M.M. *et al.* Impact of Haemophilus influenzae type b polysaccharide-tetanus protein conjugate vaccine on responses to concurrently administered diphtheria-tetanus-pertussis vaccine. *Journal of the American Medical Association* 1992; 267:673–8.

Clement International Corporation. Toxicological profile for mercury. *U.S. Department of Health and Human Services, Public Health Service, Agency for Toxic Substances and Disease* Registry. Washington, DC, 1992.

Cochi, S.L., Fleming, E.W., Hightower, A.W. *et al.* Primary invasive Haemophilus influenzae type b disease: a population based assessment of risk factors. *Journal of Pediatrics* 1986; 108:887–896.

Cochi, S.L., Preblud, S.R., Orenstein, W.A. Perspectives on the relative resurgence of mumps in the United States. *American Journal of Diseases of Children* 1988; 142:499–507.

Cody, C.L., Baraff, L.J., Cherry, J.D. *et al.* Nature and rates of adverse reactions associated with DTP and DT immunizations in infants and children. *Pediatrics* 1981; 68:650–660.

Collier, L.H., Polakoff, S., Mortimer, J. Reactions and antibody responses to reinforcing doses of adsorbed and plain tetanus vaccines. *Lancet* 1979; 1:1364.

Colville, A., Pugh, S. Mumps meningitis and measles, mumps, and rubella vaccine. *Lancet* 1992; 340:786.

Committee on Infectious Diseases, American Academy of Pediatrics. Recommendations for using pneumococcal vaccine in children. *Pediatrics* 1985; 75:1153–1158.

Committee on Infectious Diseases, American Academy of Pediatrics. Recommendations for the use of live attenuated varicella vaccine. *Pediatrics* 1995; 95:791–796.

Conflict of interest in pertussis vaccine study. *The Doctor's People* 1990; 3:4.

Corrigan, F.M., Reynolds, G.P., Ward, N.I. Aluminium and Alzheimer's disease (letter). *Lancet* 1989; 339: 268.

Coulter, H.L. *Divided Legacy: A History of the Schism in Medical Thought, Volume 3, The Conflict Between Homoeopathy and the American Medical Association: 1800–1914*. Berkeley, CA: North Atlantic Books, 1982.

Coulter, H.L. *Vaccination, Social Violence, and Criminality: The Medical Assault on the American Brain*. Berkeley, CA: North Atlantic Books, 1990.

Coulter, H.L. Review of Marie R. Griffin DTP study. Unpublished, 1990(a).

Coulter, H.L. Contribution to the discussion of connection between childhood vaccinations and neurologic disease. Submitted to the Institute of Medicine's Committee to review the adverse consequences of pertussis and rubella vaccines, 1990(b).

Coulter, H.L., Fisher, B.L. *A Shot in the Dark*. Garden City, New York: Avery Publishing Group, Inc., 1991.

Coulter, H.L., personal communication, 1995.

Crapper-McLachlan, D.R., Kruck, T.P., Lukiw, W.J., Krishnan, S.S. Would decreased aluminum ingestion reduce the incidence of Alzheimer's disease? *Canadian Medical Association Journal* 1991; 145:793–804.

Crowder, M., Higgins, H.L., Frost, J.J. Rubella susceptibility in young women of rural east Texas: 1980 and 1985. *Texas Medicine* 1987; 83:43–47.

Cummings, S., Ullman, D. *Everybody's Guide to Homeopathic Medicines*. Los Angeles: Jeremy P Tarcher, Inc., 1984.

Curtis, T. The origin of AIDS: a startling new theory attempts to answer the question "Was it an act of God or man?" *Rolling Stone* March 19, 1992.

D'Cruz, O.F., Shapiro, E.D., Spiegelman, K.N., Leicher, C.R. *et al.* Acute inflammatory demyelinating polyradiculoneuropathy (Guillain-Barré syndrome) after immunization with *Haemophilus influenzae* type b conjugate vaccine. *Journal of Pediatrics* 1989; 115:743–746.

Dacou-Voutetakis, C., Constantinidis, M. Moschos, S. *et al.* Diabetes mellitus following mumps: insulin reserve. *American Journal of Diseases of Children* 1974; 127:890–891.

Daum, R.S., Sood, S.K., Osterholm, M.T. *et al.* Decline in serum antibody to the capsule of *Haemophilus influenzae* type b in the immediate postimmunization period. *Journal of Pediatrics* 1989; 1114: 742–747.

Davidson, M., Letson, G.W., Ward. J.I. *et al.* DTP immunization and susceptibility to infectious diseases: Is there a relationship? *American Journal of Diseases of Children* 1991; 145: 750–754.

Davis, L.E., Wands, J.R., Weiss, S.A. *et al.* Central nervous system intoxication from mercurous chloride laxatives—quantitative, histochemical and ultrastructure studies. *Archives of Neurology* 1974; 30:428–431.

Deming, M.S., Jaiteh, K.O., Otten, M.W., Flagg, E.W. Epidemic poliomyelitis in The Gambia following the control of poliomyelitis as an endemic disease; II. Clinical efficacy of trivalent oral polio vaccine. *American Journal of Epidemiology* 1992; 135:393.

Desrosiers, R.C. HIV-1 origins: A finger on the missing link. *Nature* 1990; 345:288–289.

Developments with respect to the manufacture of live polio vaccine and results of utilization of killed polio vaccine. Hearing before subcommittee of the Committee on Interstate and Foreign Commerce House of Representatives (87th Congress, first session). Washington, DC: US Government Printing Office, 1961: 317–325.

Dieter, M.P., Luster, M.I., Boorman, G.A. *et al.* Immunological and biochemical responses in mice treated with mercuric chloride. *Toxicology and Applied Pharmacology* 1983; 68:218–228.

Dodge, P.R., Davis, H., Feigin, R.D. *et al.* Prospective evaluation of hearing impairment as a sequelae of acute bacterial meningitis. *New England Journal of Medicine* 1984; 311:869–874.

Dollinger, H.C., Zumkey, H., Spieker, C. *et al.* Aluminum in antacids shown to accumulate in brain and bone tissue. *Gastroenterol Obs* 1986; 5:478.

Druet, P., Druet, E., Potdevin, F. *et al.* Immune type glomerulonephritis induced by HgCl2 in the Brown Norway rat. *Annals of Immunology* 1978; 129C:777–792.

Dudley, S.F., May, P.M., O'Flynn, J.A, *Medical Research Council, Special Report Series, No. 195.* UK, 1934.

Duncan, B., Ey, J., Holberg, C.J., Wright, A.L. *et al.* Exclusive breast-feeding for at least 4 months protects against otitis media. *Pediatrics* 1993, 91:867–872.

Dunkle, L.M., Arvin, A.M., Whitley, R.J. *et al*. A controlled trial of acyclovir for chickenpox in normal children. *New England Journal of Medicine* 1991; 325:1539–1544.

Durbaca, S., Stoean, C. Investigations concerning the possibility to replace the Schick test by the passive hemagglutination reaction for evaluating the diphtheria immunity level in population. *Roumanian Archives of Microbiology and Immunology* 1992; 51: 141–146.

Dyken, P.R., Cunningham, S.C., Ward, L.C. Changing character of subacute sclerosing panencephalitis in the United States. *Pediatric Neurology* 1989; 5:339–341.

Edsall, G. Specific prophylaxis of tetanus. *Journal of American Medical Association* 1959; 171:417–427.

Edsall, G., Altman, J.S., Gaspar, A.J. Combined tetanus-diphtheria immunization of adults: use of small doses of diphtheria toxoid. *American Journal of Public Health* 1954; 44:1537–1545.

Ehrengut, W. ‹ber konvulsive Reaktionen nach Pertussis-Schutzimpfung. [Convulsive reactions after pertussis immunization.] *Deutsche Medizinische Wochenschrift* 1974; 99:2273–2279.

Eichhorn, G.L. In Katzman, R., Terry, R.D., Bick, K.L., eds. *Alzheimer's Disease: Senile Dementia and Related Disorders*. New York: Raven Press, 1978.

Eichhorn, G.L. Aging, genetics and the environment: Potential of errors introduced into genetic information transfer by metal ions. *Mech Ageing Dev* 1979; 9:291–301.

Eichhorn, G.L. Is there any relationship between aluminum and Alzheimer's disease? *Experimental Gerontology* 1993; 28:493–498.

Eisfelder, H.W. Poliomyelitis immunization—a final report. *Journal of the American Institute of Homeopathy* 1961; 54:166–167.

Elswood, B.F., Stricker, R.B. Polio vaccines and the origin of AIDS. *Research in Virology* 1993; 144:175–177.

Elswood, B.F., Stricker, R.B. Polio vaccines and the origin of AIDS. *Medical Hypotheses* 1994; 42:347–354.

English, J.M. (a) Pertussin 30—preventive for whooping cough? A pilot study. *British Homeopathic Journal* 1987; 76:61–65.

English, J.M. (b) Symptoms and treatment of whooping cough, 1980–1982. *British Homeopathic Journal* 1987; 76:66–68.

Eskola, J., Peltola, H., Takala, A.K. *et al.* Efficacy of *Haemophilus influenzae* type b polysaccharide-diphtheria toxoid conjugate vaccine in infancy. *New England Journal of Medicine* 1987; 317:717–722.

Essex, M., Kanki, P. The origins of the AIDS virus. *Scientific American* 1988; 259:64–71.

Eskola, J., Peltola, H., Takala, A.K. *et al.* Protective efficacy of the *Haemophilus influenzae* type b conjugate vaccine HbOC in Finnish infants. [Abstract #60]. *Thirtieth Interscience Conference on Antimicrobial Agents and Chemotherapy*, Atlanta, Georgia, October 1990.

Experts question need for proposed HBV requirements. *Hospital Infection Control* 1990; 17:17–28.

Facktor, M., Bernstein, R.A., Fireman, P. Hypersensitivity to tetanus toxoid. *Journal of Allergy and Clinical Immunology* 1973; 52:1–12.

Faculty review of Asian influenza. *Homeopathy* 1958; 8:115–124.

Feldman, H.M., and Michaels, R.H. Academic achievement in children ten to 12 years after *Haemophilus influenzae* meningitis. *Pediatrics* 1988; 81:339–344.

Fenichel, G.M. Neurological complications of immunization. Annals of Neurology 1982; 12:119–128.

Ferencei, M., Masar, I., Sonak, R. Comparison of the Schick test and the haemagglutination test for detection of the level of diphtheria antitoxin in the serum. *Journal of Hygiene, Epidemiology, Microbiology, and Immunology* 1969; 13: 141–148.

Fescharek, R., Quast U., Maass, G. *et al.* Measles-mumps vaccination in the FRG: an empirical analysis after 14 years of use. II. Tolerability and analysis of spontaneously reported side effects. *Vaccine* 1990; 8:446–456.

Finn, T. *Dangers of Compulsory Immunizations: How to Avoid Them Legally* New Port Richey, FL: Family Fitness Press, 1983.

Fleming, D.W., Leibenhaut, M.D., Albanes D. *et al.* Secondary *Haemophilus influenzae* type b in day-care facilities; risk factors and prevention. *Journal of the American Medical Association* 1985; 254:509–514.

Forrester, H.L., Jahnigen, D.W., LaForce, F.M. Inefficacy of pneumococcal vaccine in a high-risk population. *American Journal of Medicine* 1987; 83:425–430.

Förström, L., Hannuksela, M., Kousa, M., Kehmuskallio, E. Merthiolate hypersensitivity and vaccination. *Contact Dermatitis* 1980; 6:241–245.

Frecker, M.F. Dementia in Newfoundland: identification of a geographical isolate? In Crapper-McLachlan, D.R., Kruck, T.P., Lukiw, W.J., Krishnan, S.S. Would decreased aluminum ingestion reduce the incidence of Alzheimer's disease? *Canadian Medical Association Journal* 1991; 145:793–804.

Freed, G.L., Bordley, W.C., Clark, S.J., Konrad, T.R. Reactions of pediatricians to a new Centers for Disease Control recommendation for universal immunization of infants with hepatitis B vaccine. *Pediatrics* 1993; 91:699–702.

Freed, G.L., Bordley, W.C., Clark, S.J., Konrad, T.R. Family physician acceptance of universal hepatitis B immunization of infants. *Journal of Family Practice* 1993(a); 36:153–157.

Fulginiti, V.A. Controversies in current immunization policies and practices. *Current Problems in Pediatrics* 1976; 6:6–16.

Fulginiti, V.A. A pertussis vaccine myth dies. *American Journal of Diseases of Children* 1990; 144:860–861.

Gabriel, R. Testimony before the Committee to Review the Adverse Consequences of Pertussis and Rubella Vaccines, Institute of Medicine, May, 1990; In, Coulter, H.L. & Fisher, B.L. *A Shot in the Dark* Garden City, New York: Avery Publishing Group, Inc., 1991.

Galazka, A., Andrzejczak-Kardymowicz, B. Complication and reactions after vaccination against pertussis. *Epidemiological Review* 1972; 26:411–424.

Gale, J.L., Thapa, P.B., Bobo, J.R. *et al.* Acute neurological illness and DTP: report of a case-control study in Washington and Oregon. In Manclark, C.R., ed. Sixth International Symposium on Pertussis, Abstracts. Bethesda, Maryland: Department of Health and Human Services, 1990:228–9 (DHSS publication No. (FDA) 90–1162).

Ganiats, T.G., Bowersox, M.T. Ralph, L.P. Universal neonatal hepatitis B immunization—Are we jumping on the bandwagon too early? *Journal of Family Practice* 1993; 36:147–149.

Gao, F., Hue, L., White, A.T. *et al.* Human infection by genetically diverse SIVsm-related HIV-2 in West Africa. *Nature* 1992; 358:495–499.

Garrett, A.J., Dunham, A., Wood, D.J. Retroviruses and poliovaccines. *Lancet* 1993; 342:932–933.

Geissler, E. SV40 and human brain tumors. *Progress in Medical Virology* 1990; 37:211–222.

Gelb, L.D., Huang, J.J., Wellinghoff, W.J. Varicella-zoster virus transformation of hamster embryo cells. *Journal Gen Virology* 1980; 51:171–177.

Gershon, A.A., Steinberg, S., Galasso, G. *et al.* Live attenuated varicella vaccine in children with leukemia in remission. *Biken Journal* 1984; 27:77.

Gershon, A.A., Steinberg, S.P., Gelb, L. Live attenuated varicella vaccine use in immunocompromised children and adults. *Pediatrics* 1986; 78 (suppl):757–762.

Gershon, A.A. Live attenuated varicella vaccine. *Annals and Reviews of Medicine* 1987; 38:41–50.

Gervaix, M., Caflisch, S., Suter, A.M., Haenggeli, C.A. Guillain-Barré syndrome following immunization with *Haemophilus influenzae* type b conjugate vaccine. European *Journal of Pediatrics* 1993; 152:613–614.

Gilmartin, R.C., Jabbour, J.T., Duenas, D.A. Rubella vaccine myeloradiculoneuritis. *Journal of Pediatrics* 1972; 80:406–412.

Goffin, E., Horsmans, Y., Cornu, C. *et al.* Acute hepatitis B infection after vaccination (letter). *Lancet* 1995; 345:263.

Golden, I. A possible mechanism of homeopathic prophylaxis. *Journal of the American Institute of Homeopathy* 1989; 82: 69–76.

Golden, I. *Vaccination? A Review of Risks and Alternatives.* Aurum Healing Centre, P.O. Box 155, Daylesford, Vic. 3460, Australia, 1994.

Goldman, A.S. *et al.* Immunologic factors in human milk during the first year of lactation. *Journal of Pediatrics* 1982; 100:563.

Goto, N., Akama, K. Histopathological studies of reactions in mice injected with aluminium-adsorbed tetanus toxoid. *Microbiological Immunology* 1982; 26:1121.

Granoff, D.M., Pandey, J.P., Boies, E. *et al.* Response to immunization with *Haemophilus influenzae* type b polysaccharide-pertussis vaccine and risk of haemophilus meningitis in children with the km(1) immunoglobulin allotype. *Journal of Clinical Investigation* 1984; 74:1708–1714.

Graves, A.B., White, E., Koepsell, T.D. *et al.* The association between aluminum-containing products and Alzheimer's disease. *Journal of Clinical Epidemiology* 1990; 43:35–44.

Greenberg, M., Abrahamson, H., Cooper, H.M., Solomon, H.E. The relation between recent injections and paralytic poliomyelitis in children. *American Journal of Public Health* 1952; 42:142–152.

Griffin, M.R., Ray, W.A., Mortimer, E.A. *et al.* Risk of seizures and encephalopathy after immunization with the Diphtheria-Tetanus-Pertussis vaccine. *Journal of the American Medical Association* 1990, 263:1641–1645.

Grose, C., Spigland, I. Guillain-Barré syndrome following administration of live measles vaccine. *American Journal of Medicine* 1976; 60:441–443.

Gross, K., Combe, C., Krüger, K., Schattenkirchner, M. Arthritis after hepatitis vaccination: report of three cases. *Scandinavian Journal Rheumatology* 1995; 24:50–52.

Guess, H.A., Broughton, D.D., Melton, L.J., Kurland, L.T. Population-based studies of varicella complications. *Pediatrics* 1986; 78 (suppl):723–727.

Gunderman, J.R. Guillain-Barré syndrome: Occurrence following combined mumps-rubella vaccine. *American Journal Diseases of Children* 1973; 125:834–835.

Gupta, R.K., Relyveld, E.H. Adverse reactions after injection of adsorbed diphtheria-pertussis-tetanus (DPT) vaccine are not due only to pertussis organisms or pertussis components in the vaccine. *Vaccine* 1991; 9:699–702.

Gustafson, T.L., Lievens, A.W., Brunell, P.A. *et al.* Measles outbreak in a fully immunized secondary-school population. *New England Journal of Medicine* 1987; 316:771–774.

Hachulla, E., Houvenagel, E., Mingui, A., Vincent, G., Laine, A. Reactive arthritis after hepatitis B vaccination. *Journal of Rheumatology* 1990; 17:1250–1251.

Hadler, S.C., Francis, D.P., Maynard, J.E. *et al.* Long-term immunogenicity and efficacy of hepatitis B vaccine in homosexual men. *New England Journal of Medicine* 1986; 315:209–214.

Hahnemann, S. *The Cure and Prevention of Scarlet Fever.* Gotha: Becker Publ., 1801.

Hahnemann, S. *Organon of Medicine.* Los Angeles: J.P. Tarcher, Inc. 1982.

Hall, A.J. Hepatitis B vaccination: protection for how long and against what? Booster injections are not indicated. *British Medical Journal* 1993; 307:276–277.

Hall, C.B., Halsey, N.A. Control of hepatitis B: to be or not to be? *Pediatrics* 1992; 90:274–277.

Halperin, S.A., Barreto, L., Friesen, B., Meekison, W. Immunogenicity of a five-component acellular pertussis vaccine in infants and young children. *Archives of Pediatric and Adolescent Medicine* 1994; 148:495–502.

Haneberg, B., Matre, R., Winsnes, R. *et al.* Acute hemolytic anemia related to diphtheria-pertussis-tetanus vaccination. *Acta Paediatrica Scandinavica* 1978; 67:345–350.

Hanson, L.A., Ahlestedt, S., Andersson, B. *et al.* Protective factors in milk and the development of the immune system. *Pediatrics* 1985; 75(suppl.):172–176.

Harrison, L.H., Broome, C.V., Hightower, M.S. *et al.* A day care-based study of the efficacy of *Haemophilus influenzae* type b polysaccharide vaccine. *Journal of the American Medical Association* 1988; 260: 1413–1418.

Harrison, L.H., Broome, C.V., Hightower, M.S. *Haemophilus influenzae* type b polysaccharide vaccine: an efficacy study. *Pediatrics* 1989; 84:255–261.

Hayes, R.B., Raatgever, J.W., de Bruyn, A., Gerin, M. Cancer of the nasal cavity and paranasal sinuses, and formaldehyde exposure. *International Journal of Cancer* 1986; 37(4):487–492.

Hayflick, L., Plotkin, S.A., Norton, T.W., Koprowski, H. Preparation of poliovirus vaccines in a human fetal diploid cell strain. *American Journal of Hygiene* 1962; 75:240–258.

Hedenskog, S., Björksten, B., Blennow, M., Granström, G., Granström, M. Immunoglobulin E response to pertussis toxin in whooping cough and after immunization with a whole cell and acellular pertussis vaccine. *International Archives of Allergy and Applied Immunology* 1989; 89:156.

Helmke, K., Otten, A., Willems, W.R. *et al.* Islet cell antibodies and the development of diabetes mellitus in relation to mumps infection and mumps vaccination. *Diabetologia* 1986; 29:30–33.

Hennessen, W., Quast, U. Adverse reactions after pertussis vaccination. International Symposium on Immunization: Benefit vs. Risk Factors, Brussels. *Developments in Biological Standardization* 1979; 43:95–100.

Herroelen, L., DeKeyser, J., Ebinger, G. Central-nervous-system demyelination after immunisation with recombinant hepatitis B vaccine. *Lancet* 1991; 338:1174–1175.

Hersh, B.S., Markowitz, L.E., Hoffman, R.E. *et al.* A measles outbreak at a college with a prematriculation immunization requirement. *American Journal of Public Health* 1991; 81:360–363.

Hill, A.B., Knowelden, J. Inoculation and poliomyelitis: A statistical investigation in England and Wales in 1949. *British Medical Journal* 1950; 2:1–6.

Hinman, A.R., Koplan, J.P. Pertussis and pertussis vaccine: reanalysis of benefits, risks, and costs. *Journal of the American Medical Association* 1984; 251:3109–3113.

Hirayama, M. Measles vaccines used in Japan. *Reviews of Infectious Diseases* 1983; 5:495–503.

Hirsch, F., Kuhn, J., Ventura, M. *et al.* Autoimmunity induced by HgCl2 in Brown-Norway rats—part I: Production of monoclonal antibodies. *Journal of Immunology* 1986; 136:3272–3276.

Hirsch, R.L., Mokhtarian, F., Griffin, D.E. *et al.* Measles virus vaccination of measles seropositive individuals suppresses lymphocyte proliferation and chemotactic factor production. *Clinical Immunology and Immunopathology* 1981; 21:341–350.

Hirszel, P., Michaelson, J.H., Dodge, K. *et al.* Mercury-induced autoimmune glomerulonephritis in indbred rats—part II. Immunohistopathology, histopathology and effects of prostaglandin administration. *Survey Synth Pathological Research* 1985; 4:412–422.

Hoffman, H.J., Hunter, J.C., Damus, K. *et al.* Diphtheria-tetanus-pertussis immunization and sudden infant death: results of the National Institute of Child Health and Human Development Cooperative Epidemiological Study of Sudden Infant Death Syndrome Risk Factors. *Pediatrics* 1987; 79:598–611.

Hough, J.C. *et al.* Rubella seroconversion following immunization in a rural practice. *Journal of Family Practice* 1979; 9:587–589.

Howie, P.W. *et al.* Protective effect of breast feeding against infection. *British Medical Journal* 1990; 300:11–16.

Huet, T., Cheynier, R., Meyerhans, A. *et al.* Genetic organization of a chimpanzee lentivirus related to HIV-1. *Nature* 1990; 345:356–358.

Hulbert, T.V., Larsen, R.A., Davis, C.L., Holtom, P.D. Bilateral hearing loss after measles and rubella vaccination in an adult. *New England Journal of Medicine* 1991; 325:134.

Hull, H.F., Montes, J.M., Hays, P.C., Lucero, R.L. Risk factors for measles vaccine failure among immunized students. *Pediatrics* 1985; 76:518–523.

Hutcheson, R. DTP immunization and sudden infant death—Tennessee. *Morbidity and Mortality Weekly Report* 1979; 28:131–135.

Institute of Medicine. *An Evaluation of Poliomyelitis Vaccine Policy Options.* IOM publication 88–04, Washington, DC: National Academy of Sciences, 1988.

Institute of Medicine. *Adverse Effects of Pertussis and Rubella Vaccines.* Washington, DC: National Academy Press, 1991.

Institute of Medicine, *Adverse Events Associated with Childhood Vaccines: Evidence Bearing on Causality.* Washington, DC: National Academy Press, 1994.

Intensive Immunization Programs. *Hearings before the Committee on Interstate and Foreign Commerce, House of Representatives, 87th Congress, 2nd Session on H.R. 10541.* Washington, DC: US Government Printing Office, 1962.

Istre, G.R., Conner, J.S., Broome, C.V. *et al.* Risk factors for primary invasive *Haemophilus influenzae* disease: Increased risk from day care attendance in school age household members. *Journal of Pediatrics* 1985; 106:190–195.

Jaber, L., Shohat, M., Mimouni, M. Infectious episodes following diphtheria-pertussis-tetanus vaccination: a preliminary observation in infants. *Clinical Pediatrics* 1988; 27:491–494.

Jabbour, J.T., Duenas, D.A., Sever, J.L., Krebs, H.M. *et al.* Epidemiology of subacute sclerosing panencephalitis (SSPE) *Journal of the American Medical Association* 1972; 220:959–962.

Jacobs, J., Jimenez, L.M., Gloyd, S.S., Gale, J.L., Crothers, D. Treatment of acute childhood diarrhea with homeopathic medicine: A randomized clinical trial in Nicaragua. *Pediatrics* 1994; 93:719.

James, W. *Immunization: The Reality Behind the Myth.* Granberry, Massachusetts: Bergin & Garvey Publishers, 1988.

Jawad, A.S., Scott, D.G. Immunisation triggering rheumatoid arthritis? *Annals of Rheumatic Disease* 1989; 48:174.

Johnson, D.M. Fatal tetanus after prophylaxis with human tetanus immune globulin. *Journal of the American Medical Association* 1969; 207:1519.

Kanki, P.J., McLane, M.F., King, N.W. *et al.* Serologic identification and characterization of a macaque T-lymphotropic retrovirus closely related to HTLV-II. *Science* 1985; 228:1199–1201.

Kaplan, S.L., Fishman, M.A. Update on bacterial meningitis. *Journal of Child Neurology* 1988; 3:82–93.

Karma, P., Luotonen, J., Timonen, M. *et al.* Efficacy of pneumococcal vaccination against recurrent otitis media. Preliminary results of a field trial in Finland. *Annals of Otology, Rhinology, and Laryngology* 1980; 89:357–362.

Kazarian, E.L., Gager, W.E. Optic neuritis complicating measles, mumps, and rubella vaccination. *American Journal of Ophthalmology* 1978; 86:544–547.

Kerns, W.D., Pavkov, K.L., Donofrio, D.J. *et al.* Carcinogenicity of formaldehyde in rats and mice after long-term inhalation exposure. *Cancer Research* 1983; 43(9):4382–4392.

Khabbaz, R.F., Rowe, T., Murphey-Corb, M. *et al.* Simian immunodeficiency virus needlestick accident in a laboratory worker. *Lancet* 1992; 340:271–273.

Kilroy, A.W. Two syndromes following rubella immunization. *Journal of the American Medical Association* 1970; 214:2287–2292.

Kim-Farley, R.J., Lichfield, P.,Orenstein, W.A., Bart, K.J. *et al.* Outbreak of paralytic poliomyelitis, Taiwan. *Lancet* 1984; 2:1322–1324.

Kinnunen, E., Farkkila, M., Hovi, T., Juntunen, J., Weckstrom, P. Incidence of Guillain-Barré syndrome during a nationwide oral poliovirus vaccine campaign. *Neurology* 1989; 39:1034–1036.

Klatzo, I. *et al.* Experimental production of neurofibrillary degeneration. *Journal of Neuropathology and Experimental Neurology* 1965; 24:187.

Kleijnen, J., Knipschild, P., ter Riet, G. Clinical trials of homoeopathy. *British Medical Journal* 1991; 302:316.

Klein, A. *Trial by Fury* Charles Scribner's Sons, New York, 1972.

Koch, J., Leet, C., McCarthy, R. *et al.* Adverse events temporally associated with immunizing agents—1987 report. *Canada Diseases Weekly Report* 1989; 15:151–158.

Kopeloff, L.M. *et al.* Recurrent convulsive seizures in animals produced by immunologic and chemical means. *American Journal of Psychiatry* 1942; 98:881.

Korger, G., Quast, U, Dechert, G. Tetanusimpfung: Vertraglichkeit und Vermeidung von Nebenreaktionen. [Tetanus vaccination: tolerance and avoidance of adverse reactions.] *Klininische Wochenschrift* 1986;64:767–775.

Korn, R.F., Albrecht, R.M., Locke, F.B. The association of parenteral injections with poliomyelitis. *American Journal of Public Health* 1952; 42:153–169.

Kulenkampff, M., Schwartzman, J.S., Wilson, J. Neurological complications of pertussis inoculation. *Archives of Disease in Childhood* 1974; 49:46–49.

Kyle, W.S. Simian retroviruses, poliovaccine, and origin of AIDS. *Lancet* 1992; 339:600–601.

Lambert, H. Epidemiology of a small pertussis outbreak in Kent County, Michigan. *Public Health Rep* 1965; 80:365–369.

Landrigan, P.J., Witte, J.J. Neurologic disorder following live measles-virus vaccination. *Journal of the American Medical Association* 1973; 223:1459–1462.

Lecatsas, G., Alexander, J.J. Origins of AIDS. *Lancet* 1992; 339:1427.

Leneman, F. The Guillain-Barré syndrome. *Archives of Internal Medicine* 1966; 118:139–144.

Leung, A.K.C. Anaphylaxis due to DPT vaccine (letter). *Journal of the Royal Society of Medicine* 1985; 78:175.

Lewis, J.E. Pertussis vaccine encephalopathy (letter), *Journal of the American Medical Association* 1990; 264:2383.

License application for pertussis vaccine withdrawn in Sweden. *Lancet* 1989; I:114.

Liebling, T.; Rosenman, K.D.; Pastides, H.; *et al.* Cancer mortality among workers exposed to formaldehyde. *American Journal of Industrial Medicine* 1984; 5(6):423–428.

Lilic, D., Ghosh, S.K. Liver dysfunction and DNA antibodies after hepatitis B vaccination. *Lancet* 1994; 344:1292–1293.

Lo, K-J, Lee, S-D, Tsai, Y-T *et al.* Long-term immunogenicity and efficacy of hepatitis B vaccine in infants born to HBeAg-positive HBsAg carrier mothers. *Hepatology* 1988; 8:1647–1650.

Lockett, D. Internal memo. Advisory Committee on Immunization Practices, Centers for Disease Control. Oct. 19, 1995.

Maclaren, N., Atkinson, M. Is insulin-dependent diabetes mellitus environmentally induced? *New England Journal of Medicine* 1992; 327:348–349.

Mahurkar, S.D. *et al.* Dialysis dementia. *Lancet* 1973; 1:1412.

Makela, P.H., Sibakov, M., Herva, E., Henricksen, J. Pneumococcal vaccine and otitis media. *Lancet* 1980; 2:547–551.

Makela, P.H., Leinonen, M., Tukander, J., Karma, P. A study of the pneumococcal vaccine in prevention of clinically acute attacks of recurrent otitis media. *Review of Infectious Disease* 1981; 3:S124–S130.

Mangano, M.F., White, C.J. Varicella vaccine reflux. *Pediatrics* 1992; 89:353–354.

Marchant, D.D., Band, E., Froeschle, J.E., McVerry, P.H. Depression of anticapsular antibody after immunization with *Haemophilus influenzae* type b polysaccharide-diphtheria conjugate vaccine. *Pediatric Infectious Disease Journal* 1989; 8:508–511.

Marcuse, E.K. Why wait for DTP-E-IPV? *American Journal of Diseases of Children* 1989; 143:1006–1007.

Markowitz, L.E., Preblud, S.R., Orenstein, W.A. *et al.* Patterns of transmission in measles outbreaks in the United States, 1985–1986. *New England Journal of Medicine* 1989; 320:75–81.

Marshall, G.S., Wright, P.F., Fenichel, G.M., Karzon, D.T. Diffuse retinopathy following measles, mumps, and rubella vaccination. *Pediatrics* 1985; 76:989–991.

Martin, W.J., Ahmed, K.N., Zeng, L.C. *et al.* African green monkey origin of the atypical cytopathic 'stealth virus' isolated from a patient with chronic fatigue syndrome. *Journal of Clinical and Diagnostic Virology* 1995; 4:93–103.

Martinez, E., Domingo, P. Evans's syndrome triggered by recombinant hepatitis B vaccine. *Clinical Infectious Diseases* 1992; 15:1051.

Martyn, C.N., Osmond, C., Edwardson, J.A. *et al.* Geographical relation between Alzheimer's disease and aluminium in drinking water. *Lancet* 1989; 339: 59–62

McCloskey, B.P. The relation of prophylactic inoculations to the onset of poliomyelitis. *Lancet* 1950; 1:659–663.

McCloskey, B.P. Residual paralysis after poliomyelitis following recent inoculation. *Lancet* 1952; 1:1187–1189.

McComb, J.A., Dwyer, R.C. Passive-active immunization with tetanus immune globulin (human). *New England Journal of Medicine* 1963; 268:857–862.

McComb, J.A., Levine, L. Adult immunization: dosage reduction as a solution to increasing reactions to tetanus toxoid. *New England Journal of Medicine* 1961; 265:1152–1153.

McEwen, J. Early-onset reaction after measles vaccination: further Australian reports. *Medical Journal of Australia* 1983; 2:503–505.

McEwen, M. Should there be universal childhood vaccination against hepatitis B? *Pediatric Nursing* 1993; 19:447–452.

Medical Research Council Committee on Inoculation Procedures and Neurological Lesions. Poliomyelitis and prophylactic inoculation. *Lancet* 1956; 2:1223–1231.

Mendelsohn, R. The truth about immunizations. *The People's Doctor* April 1978, p. 1.

Meyers, J.D. Congenital varicella in term infants: Risk reconsidered. *Journal of Infectious Disease* 1974; 129:215–217.

Michel, P., Commenges, D., Dartigues, J.F. *et al.* Study of the relationship between Alzheimer's disease and aluminum in drinking water [abstr]. *Neurobiology of Aging* 1990; 11:264.

Miller, D., Madge, N., Diamond, J., Wadsworth, J., Ross, E. Pertussis immunisation and serious acute neurological illnesses in children. *British Medical Journal* 1993, 307:1171–1176.

Miller, N.Z. *Vaccines: Are They Really Safe and Effective?* Santa Fe, NM: New Atlantean Press, 1992.

Miller, N.Z. *Immuniztion, Theory vs. Reality: Exposé on Vaccinations.* Santa Fe, NM: New Atlantean Press, 1996.

Milstien, J.B., Gross, T.P., Kuritsky, J.N. Adverse reactions reported following receipt of *Haemophilus influenzae* type b vaccine: an analysis after 1 year of marketing. *Pediatrics* 1987; 80:270–274.

Mink, C.M., Sirota, N.M., Nugent, S. Outbreak of pertussis in a fully immunized adolescent and adult population. *Archives of Pediatric and Adolescent Medicine* 1994; 148:153–157.

Morgan, C.M., Cherry, J.D., Christenson, P. *et al.* A search for Bordetella pertussis infection in university students. *Clinical Infectious Diseases* 1992; 14:464–471.

Morris, J.A., Butler, H. Nature and frequency of adverse reaction following hepatitis B vaccine injection in children in New Zealand, 1985–1988. Submitted to the Vaccine Safety Committee, Institute of Medicine, Washington, DC, May 4, 1992.

Morris, K., Rylance, G. Guillain-Barré syndrome after measles, mumps, and rubella vaccine. *Lancet* 1994; 343:60.

Mortimer, E.A. Immunization against infectious disease. *Science* 1978; 200:902.

Mortimer, E.A., Kimura, M., Cherry, J.D. *et al.* Protective efficacy of the Takeda acellular pertussis vaccine combined with diphtheria and tetanus toxoids following household exposure of Japanese children. *American Journal of Diseases of Children* 1990; 144:899–904.

Moskowitz, R. The case against immunizations. *Journal of the American Institute of Homeopathy* 1983; 76:7–25.

Moskowitz, R. Postcript on immunizations: Directions for future research. *Journal of the American Institute of Homeopathy* 1985; 78: 101–104.

Moskowitz, R. Immunizations: The other side. *Mothering* 1984; 31:32–38.

Moskowitz, R. Unvaccinated children. *Mothering* 1987; 34:34–39.

Moskowitz, R. Vaccination: A sacrament of modern medicine. *Journal of the American Institute of Homeopathy* 1991; 84: 96–105.

Moxon, E.R. Modern vaccines: The scope of immunisation. The *Lancet* 1990; 335(8687):448–451.

Mühlebach-Sponer, M., Zbinden, R. da Silva, V.A., Gnehm H.E. Intrathecal rubella antibodies in an adolescent with Guillain-Barré syndrome after mumps-measles-rubella vaccination. *European Journal of Pediatrics* 1995; 154:166.

Murphy, J. *What Every Parent Should Know About Childhood Immunization,* Boston: Earth Healing Products, 1993.

Murphy, T.V., Clements, J.F., Breedlove, J.A., Hansen, E.J. *et al.* Risk of subsequent disease among day-care contacts of patients with systemic *Hemophilus influenzae* type b disease. *New England Journal of Medicine* 1987; 316:5–10.

Murphy, T.V., White, K.E., Pastor, P., Gabriel, L. *et al.* Declining incidence of *Haemophilus influenzae* type b disease since introduction of vaccination. *Journal of the American Medical Association* 1993; 269:246–248.

Myers, M.G., Beckman. C.W., Vosdingh, R.A. *et al.* Primary immunization with tetanus and diphtheria toxoids: reaction rates and immunogenicity in older children and adults. *Journal of American Medical Association* 1982; 248:2478–2480.

Nabe-Nielsen, J., Walter, B. Unilateral deafness as a complication of the mumps, measles, and rubella vaccination. *British Medical Journal* 1988; 297:489.

Naruse, H., Miwata, H., Ozaki, T., Asano, Y. *et al.* Varicella infection complicated with meningitis after immunization. *Acta Paediatrica Japonica* 1993; 35:345–347.

Nathanson, N., Langmuir, A.D. The Cutter incident: Poliomyelitis following formaldehyde-inactivated poliovirus vaccination in the United States during the spring of 1955. I. Background; II. Relationship of poliomyelitis to Cutter vaccine. *American Journal of Hygiene* 1963; 78:16–60.

Naylor, G.J., Smith, A.H.W., McHarg, A. *et al.* Raised serum aluminum concentration in Alzheimer's disease. *Trace Elements and Medicine* 1989; 6:93–95.

Nelson, N., Levine, R.J., Albert, R.E. *et al.* Contribution of formaldehyde to respiratory cancer. *Environmental Health Perspectives* 1986; 70:23–35.

Nicholson, J.K.A., Holman, R.C., Jones, B.M. *et al.* The effect of measles-rubella vaccination on lymphocyte populations and subpopulations in HIV-infected and healthy individuals. *Journal of Acquired Immune Deficiency Syndromes* 1992; 5:528–537.

Nieminen, U., Peltola, H., Syrjala, M.T. *et al.* Acute thrombocytopenic purpura following measles, mumps and rubella vaccination: A report on 23 patients. *Acta Paediatrica* 1993; 82:267–270.

Nightingale, E.O. Recommendations for a national policy on poliomyelitis vaccination. *New England Journal of Medicine* 1977; 297:249–253

Nkowane, B.M., Wassilak, S.G., Orenstein, W.A., Bart, K.J. *Vaccine-*associated paralytic poliomyelitis, United States: 1973 through 1984. *Journal of the American Medical Association* 1987; 257: 1335–1340.

Noble, G.R., Bernier, R.H., Esber, E.C. *et al.* Acellular and whole-cell pertussis vaccines in Japan: Report of a visit by US scientists. *Journal of the American Medical Association* 1987; 257:1351–1356.

Norrby, R. Polyradiculitis in connection with vaccination against morbilli, parotitis and rubella. *Lakartidningen* 1984; 81:1636–1637.

Nowak, R. HIV-2 and SIV may be the same virus. *Journal of National Institute of Health Research* 1992; 4:38–40.

Ogra, P.L., Ogra, S.S., Chiba, Y. *et al.* Rubella virus infection in juvenile rheumatoid arthritis. *Lancet* 1975; 1.

Olsen, J.H., Jensen, S.P., Hink, M. *et al.* Occupational formaldehyde exposure and increased nasal cancer risk in man. *International Journal of Cancer,* 1984; 34(5):639–644.

Oski, F.A., Naiman, J.L. Effect of live measles vaccine on the platelet count. *New England Journal of Medicine* 1966; 275:352–356.

Osterholm, M.T., Pierson, L.M., White, K.E., Libby, T.A. *et al.* The risk of subsequent transmission of *Hemophilus influenzae* type b disease among children in day care: results of a two-year statewide prospective surveillance and contact survey. *New England Journal of Medicine* 1987; 316:1–5.

Osterholm, M.T., Rambeck, J.H., White, K.E. *et al.* Lack of efficacy of Haemophilus b polysaccharide vaccine in Minnesota. *Journal of the American Medical Association* 1988; 260:1423–1428.

Osvath, P., Csorba, S., Endre, L. *et al.* IgE levels of infants with complications after pertussis vaccination. *Allergologia et Immunopathologia* 1979; 7:111–114.

Otten, A., Helmke, K., Stief, T. *et al.* Mumps, mumps vaccination, islet cell antibodies and the first manifestation of diabetes mellitus type I. *Behring Institute Mitteilungen* 1984; 75:83–88.

Ovens, H. Anaphylaxis due to vaccination in the office. *Canadian Medical Association Journal* 1986; 134:369–370.

Papers presented at discussion held at the First International Conference on Live Poliovirus Vaccines. Washington, DC: PAHO, 1959: 324–325.

Pascal, L. What happens when science goes bad. Science and Technology Analysis Working Paper No 9, *Department of Science and Technology Studies,* University of Wollongong, Australia, December 1991.

Pasko, M.T., Beam, T.R. Persistence of anti-HBs among health care personnel immunized with hepatitis B vaccine. *American Journal of Public Health* 1990; 80:590–593.

Pate, J.E. *The School Performance of Post* Haemophilus influenzae *Meningitic Children: Dallas. Final Report.* Education Resources Information Center, E.D. 067801, U.S. Office of Education, July 1, 1972.

Paterson, J., Boyd, W.E. Potency action: A preliminary study of the alteration of the Schick test by a homúopathic potency, *British Homœopathic Journal* 1941, 301–309.

Peltola, H., Kilpi, T., Anttila, M. Rapid disappearance of *Haemophilus influenzae* type b meningitis after routine childhood immunisation with conjugate vaccines. *Lancet* 1992; 340:592–594.

Perl, D.P., Brody, A.R. Alzheimer's disease: X-ray spectrometric evidence of aluminium accumulation in neurofibrillary tangle-bearing neurones. *Science* 1980; 208:297–299.

Petersen, G.M., Silimperi, D.R., Rotter, J.I. *et al.* Genetic factors in *Haemophilus influenzae* type b disease susceptibility and antibody acquisition. *Journal of Pediatrics* 1987; 110:228–233.

Philip, R.N., Reinhard, K.R., Lackman, D.B. Observations on a mumps epidemic in a "virgin" population. *American Journal of Hygiene* 1959; 69:91–111.

Pichichero, M.E., Francis, A.B., Marsocci, S.M. *et al.* Comparison of a diphtheria and tetanus toxoids and bicomponent acellular pertussis vaccine with diphtheria and tetanus toxoids and whole-cell pertussis vaccine in infants. *American Journal of Diseases of Children* 1992; 147:295–299.

Pierchella, P., Petri, H., Rüping, K.W., Stary, A. [Urticaria after H-B-Vax injection due to hypersensitivity to thiomersal (merthiolate)]

Urtikarielle Reaktion nach Injektion von H-B-Vax bei Sensibil-isierung auf Thiomersal (Merthiolat). *Allergologie* 1987; 10:97–99.

Plotkin, S. Hell's fire and varicella-vaccine safety. *New England Journal of Medicine* 1988; 318:573–575.

Poliovaccine and AIDS origin link very unlikely. *Lancet* 1992; 340:1090–1091.

Pollard, J.D., personal communication; University of Sydney, Sydney, Australia, 1993.

Pollard, J.D., Selby, G. Relapsing neuropathy due to tetanus toxoid: report of a case. *Journal of Neurological Science* 1978; 37:113–125.

Pollock, T.M., Morris, J. A 7–year survey of disorders attributed to vaccination in Northwest Thames Region. *Lancet* 1983; 1:753–757.

Popkin, B.M., Adair, L., Akin, J.S., Black, R. *et al. Pediatrics* 1990; 86:874–882.

Poullin, P., Gabriel, B. Thrombocytopenic purpura after recombinant hepatitis B vaccine. *Lancet* 1994; 344:1293.

Preblud, S.R. Varicella: complications and costs. *Pediatrics* 1986; 78 (suppl):728–735.

Read, S.J., Schapel, G.J., Pender, M.P. Acute transverse myelitis after tetanus toxoid vaccination. *Lancet* 1992; 339:1111–1112.

Recker, R.R., Blotcky, A.J., Leffler, J.A., Rack, E.P. Evidence for alu-minium absorption from the gastrointestinal tract and bone depo-sition by aluminium carbonate ingestion with normal renal function. *Journal of Laboratory and Clinical Medicine* 1977; 90:810.

Regamey, R.H. Die Tetanus-Schutzimpfung. [Tetanus immunization in *Handbook of Immunization.*] In Herrlick, A., ed. *Handbuch der Schutzimpfungen.* Berlin: Springer, 1965.

Reilly, D., Taylor, M.A., Beattie, N.G.M. *et al.* Is evidence for home-opathy reproducible? *Lancet* 1994; 344:1601.

Relihan, M. Reactions to tetanus toxoid. *Journal of the Irish Medical Association* 1969; 62:430–434.

Relyveld, E.H. Current developments in production and testing of tetanus and diphtheria vaccines. In Mizrahi, A., Hertman, I., Kling-berg, M., Kohn, A., eds. New Developments with Human and Vet-erinary *Vaccines* New York: Alan R. Liss, 1980.

Ribera, E.F., Dutka, A.J. Polyneuropathy associated with administration of hepatitis B vaccine. *New England Journal of Medicine* 1983; 309:614–615.

Rietschel, R.L., Adams, R.M. Reactions to thimerosal in hepatitis B vaccines. *Dermatologic Clinics* 1990; 8:161–164.

Roberts, S.C. Vaccination and cot deaths in perspective. *Archives of Disease in Childhood* 1987; 62:754–759.

Rosa, F.W., Sever, J.L., Madden, D.L. Absence of antibody response to simian virus 40 after inoculation with killed-poliovirus vaccine of mothers of offspring with neurologic tumors. *New England Journal of Medicine* 1988; 318:1469.

Rosa, F.W., Sever, J.L., Madden, D.L. Response to: Neurologic tumors in offspring after inoculation of mothers with killed poliovirus vaccine. *New England Journal of Medicine* 1988; 319:1226.

Ross, R.T. Varicella and remission of multiple sclerosis. *Lancet* 1991; 337:300.

Saarinen, U.M. Prolonged breast feeding as prophylaxis for recurrent otitis media. *Acta Paediatrica Scandinavica* 1982; 71:567–571.

St. Geme, J.W., George, B.L., Bush, B.M. Exaggerated natural measles following attenuated virus immunization. *Pediatrics* 1976; 57:148–150.

Salk, J., Drucker, J. Noninfectious poliovirus vaccine. In Plotkin, S.A., and Mortimer, E.A. *Vaccines*. Philadelphia: W.B. Saunders, 1988.

Santosham, M., Wolff, M., Reid, R., Hohenboken, M. *et al.* The efficacy in Navajo infants of a conjugate vaccine consisting of *Haemophilus influenzae* type b polysaccharide and Neisseria meningitidis outer-membrane protein complex. *New England Journal of Medicine* 1991; 324:1767–1772.

Saroso, J.S., Bahrawi, W., Witjaksono, H. *et al.* A controlled field trial of plain and aluminium hydroxide-adsorbed cholera vaccines in Surabaya, Indonesia, during 1973–75. *Bulletin of the World Health Organization* 1978; 56:619.

Schäfer, T., Enders, F., Przybilla, B. Sensitization to thimerosal and previous vaccination. *Contact Dermatitis* 1995; 32:114–116.

Schaffer, R. A case of oral polio vaccinosis. *Journal of the American Institute of Homeopathy* 1995; 88: 33–34.

Schaffner, W., Fleet, W.F., Kilroy, A.W. *et al.* Polyneuropathy following rubella immunization: a follow-up study and review of the problem. *American Journal of Diseases of Children* 1974; 127:684–688.

Scheibner, V. *Vaccination: The Medical Assault on the Immune System,* Blackheath, NSW, Australia, 1993.

Schick, B. Die Diphtherietoxin-Hauktreation des Menschen als Vorprobe der prophylaktischen Diphtherieheilseruminjektion. *Munchen Med. Schnschr.* 1913; 60: 2608–2610.

Schlenska, G.K. Unusual neurological complications following tetanus toxoid administration. *Journal of Neurology* 1977; 215:299–302.

Schneck, S.A. Vaccination with measles and central nervous system disease. *Neurology* 1968; 18 (Part 2):79–82.

Schoenbaum, S.C., Biano, S., Mack, T. Epidemiology of congenital rubella syndrome: The role of maternal parity. *Journal of the American Med Association* 1975; 233:151–155.

Schwartz, M. Monkey virus reportedly found in polio vaccine. *San Jose Mercury News* August 29, 1995.

Schwarz, G., Lanzer, G., List, W.F. Acute midbrain syndrome as an adverse reaction to tetanus immunization. *Intensive Care Medicine* 1988; 15:53–54.

Scott, J. The Treatment of Children by Acupuncture. Sussex, England: *Journal of Chinese Medicine* 1986.

Shaw, F.E., Graham, D.J., Guess, H.A., Milstien, J.B. *et al.* Postmarketing surveillance for neurologic adverse events reported after hepatitis B vaccination: Experience of the first three years. *American Journal of Epidemiology* 1988; 127:337–352.

Shepherd, D. *Homoeopathy in Epidemic Diseases.* Essex, England: Health Science Press, 1967.

Sell, S.H. *Haemophilus influenzae* type b meningitis: Manifestations and long-term sequelae. *Pediatric Infectious Disease Journal* 1987; 6:775–778.

Sell, S.H., Webb, W.W., Pate, J.E. *et al.* Psychological sequelae to bacterial meningitis: Two controlled studies. *Pediatrics* 1972; 49:212–217.

Shah, K., Nathanson, N. Human exposure to SV40. *American Journal of Epidemiology* 1976; 103:1–12.

Shapiro, E.D., Murphy, T.V., Wald, E.R., Brady, C.A. The protective efficacy of *Haemophilus influenzea* polysaccharide vaccine. *Journal of the American Medical Association* 1988; 260: 1419–1422.

Shasby, D.M., Shope, T.C., Downs, H., Herrmann, K.L., Polkowski, J. Epidemic measles in a highly vaccinated population. *New England Journal of Medicine* 1977; 296:585–589.

Sieber, O.F., Fulginiti, V.A. Is adult immunization more appropriate than immunization of infants? *Pediatrics* 1977; 60:562–563.

Siegel, M., Fuerst, H.T., Peress, N.S. Comparative fetal mortality in maternal virus diseases: A prospective study on rubella, measles, mumps, chickenpox, and hepatitis. *New England Journal of Medicine* 1966; 274:768–771.

Simberkoff, M.S., Cross, A.P., Al-Ibrahim, M. *et al.* Efficacy of pneumococcal vaccine in high-risk patients: Results of a Veterans Administration cooperative study. *New England Journal Med* 1986; 315:1316–1327.

Simpson, N., Simon, L., Randall, R. Parental refusal to have children immunised: extent and reasons. *British Medical Journal* 1995; 310:227.

Skudder, P.A., and McCarroll, J.R. Current status of tetanus control: Importance of human tetanus-immune globulin. *Journal of the American Med Association* 1964; 188:625–627.

Slater, D.N., Underwood, J.C.E., Durrant, T.E. *et al.* Aluminium hydroxide granulomas: Light and electron microscopic studies and x-ray microanalysis. *British Journal of Dermatology* 1982; 107:103–108.

Sloyer, J.L., Ploussard, J.H., Howie, V.M. Efficacy of pneumococcal polysaccharide vaccine in preventing acute otitis media in infants in Huntsville, Alabama. *Review of Infectious Disease* 1981; 3:S119–S123.

Smith, T. Active immunity produced by so-called balanced or neutral mixtures of diphtheria toxin and antitoxin. *Journal of Experimental Medicine* 1909; 11: 241–256.

Smits, T. The treatment and prevention of post-vaccinal disease. *Journal of the American Institute of Homeopathy* 1995; 88: 27–32.

Sood, S.K., Daum, R.S. Disease caused by *Haemophilus influenzae* type b in the immediate period after homologous immunization: immunologic investigation. *Pediatrics* 1990; 85 (4 Pt 2):698–704.

Staak, M., Wirth, E. Zur problematik anaphylaktischer Reaktionen nach aktiver Tetanus-Immunisierung. [Anaphylactic reaction following active tetanus immunization.] *Deutsche Medizinische Wochenschrift* 1973; 98:110–111.

Stayner, L., Smith, A.B., Reeve, G. *et al.* Proportionate mortality study of workers in the garment industry exposed to formaldehyde. *American Journal of Industrial Medicine* 1985; 7(3):229–240.

Stayner, L.T., Elliott, L., Blade, L. *et al.* A retrospective cohort mortality study of workers exposed to formaldehyde in the garment industry. *American Journal of Industrial Medicine* 1988; 13(6):667–681.

Stevens, C.E., Toy, P.T., Taylor, P.E., Lee, T., Yip, H. Prospects for control of hepatitis B virus infection: implications of childhood vaccination and long-term protection. *Pediatrics* 1992; 90:170–173.

Stewart, B.J.A., Prabhu, P.U. Reports of sensorineural deafness after measles, mumps, and rubella immunisation. *Archives of Diseases of Childhood* 1993; 69:153–154.

Still, C.N. Aluminum neurotoxicity and Alzheimer's disease. *Journal of the South Carolina Medical Association* 1994; November:560–564.

Storsaeter, J., Olin, P., Renemar, B. *et al.* Mortality and morbidity from invasive bacterial infections during a clinical trial of acellular pertussis vaccines in Sweden. *Pediatric Infectious Disease Journal* 1988; 7: 637–645.

Strebel P.M., Aubert-Combiescu, A., Ion-Nedelcu, N. *et al.* Paralytic poliomyelitis in Romania, 1984–1992; evidence for a high risk of vaccine associated disease and reintroduction of wild-virus infection. *American Journal of Epidemiology* 1994; 140:1111–1124.

Strebel P.M., Ion-Nedelcu, N., Baughman, A.L. *et al.* Intramuscular injections within 30 days of immunization with oral poliovirus vaccine—a risk factor for vaccine-associated paralytic poliomyelitis. *New England Journal of Medicine* 1995; 332:500–506.

Street, A.C., Weddle, T.Z. Thomann, W.R., Lundbert, E.W. *et al.* Persistence of antibody in healthcare workers vaccinated against hepatitis B. *Infection Control and Hospital Epidemiology* 1990; 11:525–530.

Sugiura, A., Yamada, A. Aseptic meningitis as a complication of mumps vaccination. *Pediatric Infectious Disease Journal* 1991; 10:209–213.

Sullivan-Bolyai, J.Z., Yin, E.K., Cox, P. *et al.* Impact of chickenpox on households of healthy children. *Pediatric Infectious Disease Journal* 1987; 6:33–35.

Sultz, H.A., Hart, B.A., Zielezny, M., Schlesinger, E.R. Is mumps virus an etiologic factor in juvenile diabetes mellitus? *Journal of Pediatrics* 1975; 86:654–656.

Suruda, A., Schulte, P., Boeniger, M. *et al.* Cytogenetic effects of formaldehyde exposure in students of mortuary science. *Cancer Epidemiology, Biomarkers and Prevention* 1993; 2(5):453–460.

Sutter, R.W., Patriarca, P.A., Brogan, S., Malankar, P.G. *et al.* Outbreak of paralytic poliomyelitis in Oman: Evidence for widespread transmission among fully vaccinated children. *Lancet* 1991; 338:715–720.

Sutter, R.W., Patriarca, P.A., Suleiman, A.J.M. *et al.* Attributable risk of DTP (diphtheria and tetanus toxoids and pertussis vaccine) injection in provoking paralytic poliomyelitis during a large outbreak in Oman. *Journal of Infectious Disease* 1992; 165:444–449.

Swartz, T.A., Klingberg, W., Goldwasser, R.A. *et al.* Clinical manifestations, according to age, among females given HPV-77 duck rubella vaccine. *American Journal of Epidemiology* 1971; 94:246–251.

Swenberg, J.A., Kerns, W.D., Mitchell, R.I. *et al.* Induction of squamous cell carcinomas of the rat nasal cavity by inhalation exposure to formaldehyde vapor. *Cancer Research* 1980; 40(9):3398–3402.

Tager, A. Preliminary report on the treatment of recurrent herpes simplex with poliomyelitis vaccine (Sabin's). *Dermatologica* 1974; 149:253–255.

Taylor Reilly, D., Taylor Reilly, M., McSharry, C., Aitchinson, T. Is homoeopathy a placebo response? Controlled trial of homoeopathic potency, with pollen in hayfever as model. *Lancet* 1986; 2:881.

Teele, D.W., Pelton, S.I., Klein, J.O. Bacteriology of acute otitis media unresponsive to initial antimicrobial therapy. *Journal of Pediatrics* 1981; 98:537–539.

Tejani, A., Dobias, B., Sambursky, J. Long-term prognosis after *H. influenzae* meningitis: Prospective evaluation. *Developmental Medicine in Child Neurology* 1982; 24:338–343.

Thompson, G.R., Weiss, J.J., Shillis, J.L., Brackett, R.G. Intermittent arthritis following rubella vaccination: a three year follow-up. *American Journal of Diseases of Children* 1973; 125:526–530.

Thompson, N.P., Montgomery, S.M., Pounder, R.E., Wakefield, A.J. Is measles vaccination a risk factor for inflammatory bowel disease? *Lancet* 1995; 345:1071–1073.

Thompson, N.P., Montgomery, S.M., Pounder, R.E., Wakefield, A.J. Measles vaccination as a risk factor for inflammatory bowel disease (letter). *Lancet* 1995(a); 345:1364.

Tingle, A.J., Pot, C.H., Chantler, J.K. Prolonged arthritis, viraemia, hypogammaglobulinaemia, and failed seroconvesion following rubella immunisation (letter). *Lancet* 1984; 1:1475–1476.

Tingle, A.J., Chantler, J.K., Pot, K.H. *et al.* Postpartum rubella immunization: association with development of prolonged arthritis, neurological sequelae, and chronic rubella viremia. *Journal of Infectious Diseases* 1985; 152:606–612.

Tingle, A.J., Allen, M., Petty, R.E. *et al.* Rubella-associated arthritis. I Comparative study of joint manifestations associated with natural rubella infection and RA 27/3 rubella immunisation. *Annals of the Rheumatic Diseases* 1986; 45:110–114.

Topaloglu, H., Berker, M., Kansu, T. *et al.* Optic neuritis and myelitis after booster tetanus toxoid vaccination (letter). *Lancet* 1992; 339:178–179.

Toraldo, R., Tolone, C., Catalanotti, P. *et al.* Effect of measles-mumps-rubella vaccination on polymorphonuclear neutrophil functions in children. *Acta Paediatrica* 1992; 81:887–890.

Torch, W. Diphtheria-pertussis-tetanus (DTP) immunization: A potential cause of the sudden infant death syndrome (SIDS). *Neurology* 1982; 32:A169.

Torch, W. Characteristics of diphtheria-pertussis-tetanus (DPT) post-vaccinal deaths and DPT-caused sudden infant death syndrome (SIDS): a review (abstract). *Neurology* 1986; 36 (Suppl. 1):148.

Tosti, A., Melino, M., Bardazzi, F. Systemic reactions due to thimerosal. *Contact Dermatitis* 1986; 15:187–188.

Tosti, A., Guerra, L., Bardazzi, F. Hyposensitizing therapy with standard antigenic extracts: An important source of thimerosal sensitization. *Contact Dermatitis* 1989; 20:173–176.

Trevisani, F., Gattinara, G.C., Caraceni, P., Bernardi, M. *et al.* Transverse myelitis following hepatitis B vaccination. *Journal of Hepatology* 1993; 19:317–318.

Troen, P., Kaufman, S.A., Katz, K.H. Mercuric bichloride poisoning. *New England Journal of Medicine* 1951; 244:459–463.

Uhari, M., Rantala, H., Niemala, M. Cluster of childhood Guillain-Barré cases after an oral poliovaccine campaign. *Lancet* 1989; 2:440–441.

Vadheim, C.M., Greenberg, D.P., Partridge, S., Jing, J. *et al.* Effectiveness and safety of an *Haemophilus influenzae* type b conjugate vaccine (PRP-T) in young infants. *Pediatrics* 1993; 92:272–279.

Vadheim, C.M., Greenberg, D.P., Eriksen, E., Hemenway, L. *et al.* Eradication of *Haemophilus influenzae* type b disease in Southern California. *Archives Pediatric and Adolescent Medicine* 1994; 148:51–56.

Vaughan, T.L., Strader, C., Davis, S., Daling, J.R. Formaldehyde and cancers of the pharynx, sinus and nasal cavity: II. Residential exposures. *International Journal of Cancer* 1986; 38:685–688.

Vautier, G., Carty, J.E. Acute sero-positive rheumatoid arthritis occurring after hepatitis vaccination. *British Journal of Rheumatology* 1994; 33:991.

Vogt, T. Water quality and health—a study of a possible relationship between aluminium in drinking water and dementia. Sosiale og okonomiske studier 61:1–99. Oslo: Central Bureau of Statistics of Norway, 1986.

Waisbren, B.A. A commentary regarding personal observations of demyelinizing disease caused by viral vaccines, borrelia infections, and proteolytic enzymes. Paper submitted to the Vaccine Safety Committee, Institute of Medicine, Washington, DC, August 11, 1992.

Wakefield, A.J., Ekbom, A., Dhillon, A.P. *et al.* Crohn's disease: pathogenesis and persistent measles virus infection. *Gastroenterology* 1995; 108:911–916.

Walker, A.M., Jick, H., Perera, D.R. *et al.* Diphtheria-tetanus-pertussis immunization and sudden infant death syndrome. *Am Journal of Public Health* 1987; 77:945–951.

Walker, A.M. Does pertussis vaccine cause sudden infant death? Presentation for Institute of Medicine Workshop on Possible Adverse Consequences of Pertussis and Rubella Vaccines, Washington, DC, May 14, 1990. Unpublished.

Ward, J. Newer *Haemophilus influenzae* type b vaccines and passive prophylaxis. *Pediatric Infectious Disease Journal* 1987; 6:799–803.

Ward, J., Brenneman, G., Letson, G.W., Heyward, W.L. Alaska *H. Influenzae* Vaccine Study Group. Limited efficacy of a *H. influenzae* type b conjugate vaccine in Alaska Native infants. *New England Journal of Medicine* 1990; 323:1381–1387.

Watson, B.M., Piercy, S.A., Plotkin, S.A., Starr, S.E. Modified chickenpox in children immunized with the Oka-Merck varicella vaccine. *Pediatrics* 1993; 91:17–22.

Weibel, R.E., Stokes, J., Buynak, E.B., Hilleman, M.R. Influence of age on clinical response to HPV-77 duck rubella vaccine. *Journal of American Medical Association* 1972; 222:805–807.

Weiner, L.B., Corwin, R.M., Nieburg, P.I., Feldman, H.A. A Measles outbreak among adolescents. *Journal of Pediatrics* 1977; 90:17–20.

Weiss, K.B., Gergen, P.J., Hodgson, T.A. An economic evaluation of asthma in the United States. *New England Journal of Medicine* 1992; 326: 862–866.

Weller, T.H. Varicella and herpes zoster: changing concepts of the natural history, control, and importance of a not-so-benign virus. *New England Journal of Medicine* 1983; 309:1362–1367.

Wentz, K.R., Marcuse, E.K. Diphtheria-tetanus-pertussis vaccine and serious neurologic illness: an updated review of the epidemiologic evidence. *Pediatrics* 1991; 87:287–297.

Werne, J., Garrow, I. Fatal anaphylactic shock: occurrence in identical twins following second injection of diphtheria toxoid and pertussis antigen. *Journal of American Medical Association* 1946; 131:730–735.

Wessel, D. Long incubation: A vaccine to prevent chickenpox is near; now, will it be used? *Wall Street Journal* Jan. 16, 1985:1.

White, F. Measles vaccine associated encephalitis in Canada. *Lancet* 1983, 2:683–684.

White, W.G., Barnes, G.M., Barker, E. *et al.* Reactions to tetanus toxoid. *Journal of Hygiene* 1983; 71:283–297.

Williams, W.W., Hickson, M.A., Kane, M.A. *et al.* Immunization policies and vaccine coverage among adults: the risk for missed opportunities. *Annals of Internal Medicine* 1988; 108:616–625.

Wyatt, H.V. Provocation of poliomyelitis by multiple injections. *Transactions of the Royal Society of Tropical Medicine & Hygiene* 1985; 79:355–358.

Yamanishi, K., Matsunaga, Y., Ogino, T., Lopetegui, P. Biochemical transformation of mouse cells by varicella-zoster virus. *Journal Gen Virology* 1981; 56:421–430.

Zupanska, B., Lawkowicz, W., Gorska, B. *et al.* Autoimmune haemolytic anaemia in children. *British Journal of Haematology* 1976; 34:511–520.

Index

About the Author

PHOTO BY MICHELE CHANDLER

Randall Neustaedter has practiced homeopathic medicine for over twenty years, specializing in child health care. He is also a licensed acupuncturist who received his Doctorate in Oriental Medicine in Hong Kong in 1983. The author of *Homeopathic Pediatrics* and *The Immunization Decision,* he is a regular contributor to homeopathic medical literature. His medical practice integrates homeopathy and Traditional Chinese Medicine. He lives and works in the San Francisco Bay Area.